FULL DISCLOSURE

DR. GARY L. GLUM

FULL DISCLOSURE

SILENT WALKER
PUBLISHING
LOS ANGELES

All of the events and characters depicted in this book are non-fictional

 Published in the United States by Silent Walker Publishing, Los Angeles.

ISBN 0-9620364-1-2

Manufactured in the United States of America
Typography and binding design by Silent Walker Publishing

First Edition

Dedicated to
my friend

Red Feather

INTRODUCTION

A few years ago, I was approached by a man who was dying of cancer. His doctors had written him off. They had told him there was nothing they could do; he was terminal. After we got to know each other, he decided for reasons of his own to confide in me the dark secrets that he knew as a result of his career in some very dark places. He knew the dark truth about our worst nightmare, he said: The AIDS virus was created by man. Intentionally. The AIDS epidemic was designed with specific goals in mind and carried out according to plan.

Like everyone else, I'd heard that speculation. And I knew that anyone who indulged in it was likely to be dismissed as a nut case. How could anyone believe such a monstrous fantasy? It made no sense. It was beyond imagination. But this man was very sane. He was a solid professional, whose connections were at high levels in several countries. He was not indulging in speculation. He knew what he was talking about. He knew the names and the numbers. He knew where some of the work was done. He knew the answers to the questions: How? And why? He knew many of the details. He knew where to look for the rest.

I've spent the years since then pursuing the truth about the

AIDS epidemic. It was not a pleasant experience. This is a truth that we were never supposed to know. It was supposed to remain a secret. Forever. To my surprise, I discovered that a lot of people—scientists, doctors, government intelligence agents, even some politicians—know parts of the story and are willing to talk about it, if their anonymity is protected.

A few of them have gone public, most notably, Dr. John Seale in England, but the press has generally ignored them—or ridiculed them. The press, after all, has its reputation to uphold. It would not want to risk dismissal as a nut case by flirting with dangerous truths. Better to accept the conventional wisdom as passed down by government officials who are, in the words of one observer, "paid a salary to tell lies to the American people."

That's part of the AIDS tragedy. Millions are dying around the world and millions more will probably die before the public even becomes aware of what has really happened to us in the last fifteen years—and why it has happened. *Full Disclosure* answers those questions: How? And why? I offer it in the cause of public awareness. I trust that it will inspire others to pursue the truth. Because the truth is our only hope.

CHAPTER ONE

"It is entirely plausible that the AIDS epidemic was started in the U.S. deliberately. Few people would need to know of the plan, and the actions of one person would be sufficient to ignite the epidemic. Maximum effectiveness would require that the introduction of effective means of stopping the virus was blocked for as long as possible, by a carefully planned and sustained campaign of disinformation. The special problem of the release of an AIDS-like virus is that it opens up a Pandora's Box, but it is naive to believe that nobody would be willing to do so."

—Dr. John Seale
Member of the Royal College of Medicine, London
Journal of the Royal Society of Medicine
September 1988 (Volume 81 pp 537-539)

For the sake of his conservative audience of British physicians, Dr. Seale was understating his own conclusion based on his research into the AIDS epidemic. What he was trying to tell them, in the gentlest way possible, was this: the deliberate introduction of the AIDS virus into mankind is exactly what has happened.

Dr. Seale was one of the first medical doctors to break the code of silence about the true cause of the AIDS epidemic. His paper hit the British medical profession like a bombshell, but few among the general public became aware of the explosion. The media ignored the story. "The scale of the deception and the misinformation has been astonishing," Dr. Seale wrote. "The virus has the properties of a skilled, devious, hidden and implacable invader with the capacity and willingness to kill every man, woman and child on earth. Dissemination of the virus is being actively encouraged by some who wish to destroy our society."

What we've come to believe about AIDS is what we've been conditioned to believe—by the carefully planned and sustained campaign of disinformation: that AIDS is a plague of nature; but not to worry, it will spare most of us, if we behave ourselves. We've been conditioned to believe that after eons of human life, nature—suddenly—about fifteen years ago, created the most deadly virus since the Black Plague of the Middle Ages—and unleashed it upon millions of Africans and Brazilians and Haitians and American homosexuals and drug addicts, and a small, unfortunate number of white heterosexuals and innocent victims of tainted blood transfusions. We've been conditioned to believe that AIDS is, so to speak, an act of God.

But it isn't. AIDS was not an accident of nature. Nature had nothing to do with AIDS. The virus is a weapon of man—against man. It is a weapon of war, deliberately created inside the top-secret U.S. Chemical and Bacteriological Warfare laboratories at Fort Detrick, Maryland and Los Alamos, New Mexico—the same government installation where the U.S., fifty years ago, developed the nuclear bombs that were dropped on Japan. The genesis of the AIDS virus can be traced back even further to a very rich and very private and virtually unknown scientific laboratory in Cold Spring Harbor, Long Island. If you know the truth about Cold Spring Harbor, you will know the truth about AIDS.

I will tell you as much of that as I know. The truth is so horrifying that it is almost impossible to believe: that officials inside our own government, backed by some of the most powerful families on earth, could be guilty of genocide. But enough proof of that truth has already leaked out to persuade many knowledgeable researchers, such as Dr. Seale, to come forth publicly with what they've learned. In a strange way, the truth behind the AIDS epidemic isn't even such a closely held secret anymore. The media has chosen to ignore it. Certainly no politician has dared utter one word about it publicly. But scientists and doctors and government intelligence agents and political leaders all around the world are aware of bits and pieces of it. They are just waiting for the public to catch on.

In the meantime, most of them want nothing to do with exposing the truth; they are too frightened to discuss it with anybody but their most trusted friends. A few of them, like Dr. Seale, are trying to expose it. "Every biological scientist who has dispassionately studied the virus and the epidemic," Dr. Seale has written, "knows that the origins of the virus could lie in the development of modern biology, just as the origins of the nuclear bomb with modern physics. Most biological scientists have not yet come to terms with the terrible truth and have developed various neurotic reactions to cope with it. Many have developed a selective denial of reality and genuinely cannot see what is happening. Most who see it keep quiet, but increasing numbers are talking privately though they still lack the moral courage to speak out in public. They still hope it is a nightmare which will vanish with tomorrow's dawn. Some who know perfectly well what is happening are deliberately fudging scientific data to keep the heat off them and fellow scientists of their molecular biological 'club.' "

The doctors and scientists and intelligence agents who are risking their reputations—and their careers and their lives—to bring forth the truth are the real heroes of the AIDS epidemic. If the public ever learns enough to demand legal retribution against those responsible for AIDS—and force the government into employing proper methods of epidemic control that will help to spare those as yet uninfected, and their children and grandchildren—they are the ones who will go down in history as saviours of much, if not all, of mankind.

I don't pretend to know the whole story. I don't believe anybody who wasn't involved in the creation and spread of AIDS to its carefully selected target groups knows the whole story. But I know enough to sketch the outline that follows. Perhaps the most important point to make is that AIDS did not happen by accident—any more than it did by nature. Nor is it the result of an insane plot by some deranged scientist—or even a small team of deranged scientists. AIDS was the result of a decades-long research program carried out in Chemical and Bacteriological Warfare labs in this country and others. For those involved, it is a triumph of science and the answer to what they regard as the planet's most pressing problem: population control.

AIDS is the perfect biological weapon. It can be confined with some degree of success to certain specific groups, and since the incubation period can be more than seven years, millions can be infected before the first person in the chain displays any symptoms. When you really understand the background to AIDS, you see that it is not only believable; it is utterly logical. Once science was far enough advanced in biotechnology to create and destroy life through microscopic manipulations of cells, it was inevitable that this type of bacteriological weapon—this plague, which is capable of killing every man, woman and child on earth—was inevitable. Just as it was inevitable that nuclear bombs would be dropped once physicists had split the atom in a world at war.

CHAPTER TWO

The government's secret branches that develop biochemical weapons have a long history of criminal behavior. AIDS is merely the most lethal of their nefarious projects. Thirty years ago, in the early 1960s, as part of their "MK-Ultra" program to develop powerful methods of mind control, CIA officers went into bars and cocktail parties all across America—even ran a brothel in the Bay Area, complete with one-way mirrors and cameras—and secretly laced innocent people's drinks with a potent new drug they were testing. It was called LSD. America can thank the CIA for the explosion of LSD use—with all the havoc and grief it has wreaked—since the 1960s. They weren't even above testing it on unsuspecting U.S. military officers, at least one of whom, in his chemically induced madness, committed suicide—and it was years before his own family discovered the truth of what their government had done to one of its own officers.

It's been well-documented that from 1949-1969 the Army used the public as guinea pigs for its bacteriological tests in several American cities—and on a large scale. The bacteria was sprayed through the North Terminal at Washington National

Airport and on the walls of New York City's subways. The bacteria was also released in Florida, California and Alaska. At one site on the Pennsylvania Turnpike, passing cars and trucks were sprayed with the bacteria. The Army just wanted to find out what its new bacteria would do to people.

As this book was nearing publication, the details of the Army's Chemical and Bacteriological Warfare experimentation on American cities continued to leak out. In this case, more than forty years later. I quote from the National Edition of the *New York Times*, June 10, 1994. An obscure story in a few paragraphs at the bottom of page nine: "Minneapolis Called Toxic Spraying Site," the headline read. The story read: "In a 1953 cold war experiment, the Army sprayed clouds of toxic material over Minneapolis dozens of times and may have caused miscarriages and still-births, a public television station here has reported.

"The sprayings in Minneapolis and other cities were described then as part of an effort to develop an aerosol screen to protect Americans from fallout in case of an atomic attack . . . The material sprayed in Minneapolis was zinc cadmium sulfide, a suspected carcinogen, and the Army was actually testing how chemicals would disperse during biological warfare, the station reported.

"One of the sites sprayed in Minneapolis was a public elementary school where former students have reported an unusual number of stillbirths and miscarriages. . . .

"In its report, the station quoted experts as saying zinc cadmium sulfide was toxic and might cause cancer. It said it was sprayed 61 times in four parts of Minneapolis, from generators in the rear of trucks or from rooftops.

"One former student of the sprayed school told the station that of her three children, one had Down's syndrome, another was profoundly retarded and a third had a learning disability."

This was all done in the cause of Chemical and Bacteriological Warfare. We've read about its existence. It appears in the news every once in a while. The Soviets were said to possess a nightmarish capacity. President Nixon made headlines around the world when he announced he would seek a ban on it. (Nothing happened.) It made big headlines when herds of sheep mysteriously fell over dead in their fields near the Army's secretive CAB lab at Dugway, Utah. The Army, of course, lied through its teeth and denied any knowledge of what might have happened, but the public discovered years later that the wind changed on a day when they were testing one of their deadly airborne toxins.

The post-Watergate investigations, more than a decade after the CIA's MK-Ultra mind control programs, finally brought forth the shocking news that the CIA was drugging thousands of unsuspecting Americans—and the scientist in charge, Sid Gottlieb, fled to India rather than answer to Congress. Or face prison.

Intelligence sources have informed me that he was also involved in the program to develop a virus, then unnamed, that would kill by destroying the body's immune system. That's the one that became known as AIDS. It may seem unimaginable to an ordinary citizen that the government could be deliberately working on a virus to destroy the human immune system. But why not? Probed by a Senator in front of TV cameras about whether the CIA had ever considered some exquisitely exotic killing device, former CIA director Richard Helms responded coldly: "Senator, we consider everything." How much of a leap of imagination was it for someone like Gottlieb, who'd spent years on the government payroll testing—on his fellow citizens—secret and dangerous drugs that created madness and death, to work on a lethal virus?

The true stories about Saddam Hussein gassing thousands of Kurds to death—and speculation that he might employ chemical and bacteriological weapons against U.S. troops—were used to whip up American war fever after the Iraqi invasion of Kuwait. And then it goes away until next time. The whole subject of Chemical and Bacteriological Warfare just disappears from the media's—and the public's—radar screen. It's as if amnesia sets in.

Meanwhile, every day for the last several decades, many thousands of the world's top scientists and engineers and lab technicians, operating with enormous secret budgets, have devoted their talents to exploiting the microscopic secrets of nature as a weapon to kill, maim, disable or control human beings.

Item: Under a CIA-funded program, neurotoxins were developed that could attack the nervous sytem and paralyze people who received them either through freeze-dried, aerosol or other means. Such toxins were manufactured from complex proteins that were subdivided to isolate certain segments or "active sites." The goal of that program was to find a way in which large areas—even entire urban areas—could be targeted to dull people's decision-making processes and instill a false sense of euphoria. Imagine how effective this would be in "neutralizing" enemy camps—whether they were soldiers from another country or political activists within our own.

The CIA can take you up. But they can also bring you down. Using its own Chemical and Bacteriological Warfare facilities, the CIA developed small, almost weightless, peptides that acted as sedatives. With slight modifications, based on DNA research, organisms were created which could produce toxic proteins capable of instilling either terrible fear or erratic behavior and bizarre actions not characteristic of the individuals in the targeted group. Imagine the effects of this toxin released in aerosol form in a political forum gathered in a small room—or even a large meeting hall. And who would ever know that this new "technique" of disruption had been employed by the government?

Literally hundreds of studies were done for the CIA in the area of neuropharmacology, particularly in the area of intercellular communications-neurotransmitters. The idea was to find a chemical substance that could be easily administered through aerosols to interfere and "mix up" neurotransmitters. (A substance was isolated which has a special "affinity" for a specific cell which required only pico or nanograms to entirely disable the "target" in a very selective way and without arousing suspicions.)

Item: Freeze-dried and microencapsulization techniques developed by the U.S. Army (primarily at Fort Detrick and Los Alamos) since 1967 were successful in creating a product that reduces toxicity to the agent handling the material and allows dissemination on impact and a sustained release. Using these techniques, the U.S. government now has the capability of delivering any virus to any unsuspecting person or group.

According to documents in the possession of certain U.S. Senate intelligence oversight committees, even the Bubonic Plague virus can now be aerosolized and used on specified targets, either here or abroad. One little known detail of the Persian Gulf War is that the CIA made several unsuccessful attempts to infect Iraqi dictator Saddam Hussein with a rapidly acting type of Legionnaire's virus.

Question: How, then, can we know if someone who died of "natural causes" was actually the target of this type of weapon? Answer: We can't. For years, spy novelists wrote about agents who were killed by "heart attack," through the use of curare-tipped instruments. A little pin prick—the tip of an umbrella into a calf—and you're dead. But that's long since obsolete; no self-respecting spy novelist would dream of using a curare pinprick in his story anymore than any government agent would use it in real life. It's too easily detectable by new technology and the story has been told too many times by the John LeCarre's of the world. The agents and the spy novelists have advanced way beyond that.

Item: A new synthetic "heroin" was produced. It is four times stronger than real heroin. Freeze dried, encapsulated and put into aerosol form, it was then sprayed into known hangouts of drug addicts over a period of six months. The report on this experiment called it "highly effective." This new heroin substitute was then mixed with regular heroin and allowed to be distributed through the illicit drug network.

Those unfortunate enough to "try" heroin for the first time containing this additive were instantly addicted for life. Using the same technology, the AIDS virus was mixed into batches of heroin and cocaine—to speed up the epidemic among drug addicts and allow the mainstream population to believe that AIDS was not something they had to worry about. Those damned gays and drug abusers were bringing this plague upon themselves!

What emerged from the Fort Detrick tests helps to explain the rapid spread of AIDS among drug abusers. Since only a small minority of drug abusers "shoot" their drugs, contaminated needles could in no way be the sole cause for the bombshell of AIDS which hit drug abusers. That's like saying that the HIV virus was carried from Haiti and spread among homosexuals in America. But this would not account for the 9000-power spread of the disease.

According to intelligence documents, the HIV virus freeze-dried and encapsulated in "mainline" heroin shots and mixed with cocaine for "snorting" would have an instantaneous effect through the nasal membranes, ensuring that the inhaler would come down with AIDS in due course.

Fort Detrick researchers actually did a paper on this subject. If it hasn't been destroyed, it's still in their highly classified files. But only a miracle would ever bring it forth for public scrutiny. Other intelligence reports do, however, indicate that batches of AIDS-infected drugs were released "onto the market."

The AIDS virus is but one of many biochemical tools of destruction our government has created. If the public knew how many billions of tax dollars have been spent to create and produce and stockpile these microscopic weapons of mass destruction, they wouldn't even be shocked to discover that a virus that destroys the human immune system has become an operational part of their vast arsenal.

The implications are not difficult to imagine. Are you a member of a target group that the government—or some renegade group in the government—deems undesirable? Here's what's in store: Zbigniew Brzezinski wrote in *The Technotronic Era* in 1972, "At the same time the capacity to assert social and political control over the individual will vastly increase. It will soon be possible to assert almost continuous control over every citizen, and to maintain individual files containing even the most personal behavior of every citizen, in addition to the customary data.

"These files will be subject to instantaneous retrieval by the authorities. Power will gravitate into the hands of those who control information . . . This will encourage tendencies through the next several decades toward a technotronic era, a dictatorship, leaving less and less room for political procedures as we now know them. Finally, looking ahead to the turn of the century, the possibility of biochemical and mind control and genetic tinkering with man, including beings which will function like men and reason like them, could give rise to some difficult questions."

A generation ago, Brzezinski's ideas might have sounded to ordinary people like the rantings of some lunatic fringe case. But he knew what he was talking about. He was a true insider. Five years after he wrote those words, he was named National Security Adviser to President Carter. If a person of that stature dared to say the above publicly, just try to imagine what they were saying to each other privately. At the moment Brezezinski wrote about future "genetic tinkering with man," the research was already progressing on the creation of a virus designed to destroy the human immune system.

As we approach the turn of the century, just as he predicted, those "difficult questions" are being answered secretly in Chemical and Bacteriological Warfare laboratories in the West and Russia. It's not even difficult to understand why. Brzezinski has already told us: It's about control. Mind control. Political control. And, ultimately: Population control.

CHAPTER THREE

AIDS is the weapon of a powerful segment of society whose spiritual forefathers date back centuries. The epidemic is the culmination of the intellectual and spiritual tradition of some of the richest and most powerful people alive, many of them famous and respected figures from families whose names are household words and held in high esteem by the public. Their indifference —or contempt—for the lives of common humanity should not come as a surprise, nor be hard to believe.

Since at least the height of British colonial domination of the world, there has been a potent strain of thinking among "aristocrats" about superior races (white, English speaking, educated and rich) and inferior races (white or black or colored, uneducated and poor). The entire British colonial system was based on the ruthless domination by a few of the "superior" over vast numbers of the "inferior."

America itself was founded in rebellion against that domination. The American Revolution was an overthrow of those old ideas about who should rule—and how. And then the new Americans turned right around and did the same thing to their own "inferiors," allowing slavery for blacks and committing genocide against Native Americans with a rapacity that would have gratified the most ruthless British colonialists.

Philosophers revered as great thinkers by the British aristocrats of those centuries openly expressed their views that the inferior peoples of the planet must not be allowed to increase sufficiently in numbers to use up the earth's precious natural resources and, eventually, to overrun by sheer numbers the existing political and economic system.

The most prominent 18th Century spokesman for the British East India Company policies of global genocide was the economist Adam Smith. His book, *The Wealth of Nations*, is still required reading in college economics classes. He wrote several works on forced population reduction, the most notable being *The Treatise of Human Nature* and *The Theory of Moral Sentiments*, in which he placed mankind on the level of animals.

Smith's ideas were advanced in the 19th Century by philosophers as prominent as Thomas Malthus, another high-ranking employee of the British East India Company. To the acclaim of the British upper classes, Malthus actually wrote in the mid-1800's: "All children who are born, beyond what would be needed to keep up the population to a desired level, must necessarily perish, unless room be made for them by the death of grown persons . . . We should facilitate, instead of desperately trying to impede, the operation of nature in producing this mortality, and if we dread the all too often visitation of the horrid form of famine, we should sedulously encourage the other forms of destruction which we compel nature to use."

Malthus' modest proposals included that the poor be educated into habits of filth rather than cleanliness and that poor villages should be built "near stagnant pools and particularly encourage settlements in marshy and unwholesome situations." And he encouraged that restraint be enforced upon those misguidedly benevolent men who would try to protect the poor from contagious diseases.

Malthus was a respected writer of his era, and though not one American in a thousand has read his work since some boring college class, his name remains famous. His writings were eminent enough to be responsible for the invention of a word that remains in our language even now: Malthusian. Meaning: "Of or pertaining to the theory of Thomas Malthus that population tends to increase faster than food supply, with inevitably disastrous results unless the increase in population can be checked."

Inevitably disastrous results unless the increase in population can be checked. Precisely. And in one sentence, the meaning of "Malthusian" captures perfectly what the AIDS epidemic is really all about: Population control. Malthusian philosophy was heralded in the 20th Century by esteemed British writers who included H. G. Wells (of "War of the Worlds" fame) and Lord Bertrand Russell. Near the end of his long life, Lord Russell won acclaim among antiwar activists for his outspoken opposition to American involvement in Vietnam. But what they didn't know was that he just thought war was a horribly messy and inefficient way to kill people. Not to mention the property destruction and expensive munitions.

Throughout his career, Lord Russell spoke of the aristocratic aspiration toward a more refined form of genocide. In *The Impact of Science on Society*, he made it clear what they had in mind: "I do not pretend that birth control is the only way in which population can be kept from increasing. There are others, which, one must suppose, opponents of birth control would prefer. War, as I remarked a moment ago, has hitherto been disappointing in this respect, but perhaps bacteriological war may prove effective. If a Black Death could be spread throughout the world once in every generation, survivors could procreate freely without making the world too full. There would be nothing in this to offend the conscience of the devout or to restrain the ambition of nationalists. This state of affairs might be somewhat unpleasant, but what of it. Really high-minded people are indifferent to suffering, especially that of others."

But of course. How else to run an empire? In 1953, when Lord Russell's book was published, there was very little public knowledge of bacteriological warfare. Yet he spoke of it knowingly and lovingly, and he clearly indicated that poor nations would be targeted.

That virulent strain of thought continues—and reaches to the top. In 1962, the CIBA foundation held a symposium, "Man and His Future," at which the keynote speaker was Francis Krick. His favored tactics of population control included putting a chemical that would cause sterility in the water supplies of those nations he judged as "not fit to have children." Other nations deemed fit would be given a license to purchase an antidote.

"This approach may run against Christian ethics," he said in a nice touch of understatement, "but I do not see why people should have a right to have children. We might be able to achieve remarkable results after twenty or thirty years by limiting reproduction to genetically superior couples."

He talked about the benefits that could come to a country that "improved its population on a grand scale." What type of people was Frick talking about? A study of his work leaves no doubt that "limiting reproduction to genetically superior couples," as he wished to do, would exclude Negroes, Jews, Gypsies and the Asian races. The year was not 1939 but 1962, and the country was not Nazi Germany, but the United States of America. These were not the musings of a deranged madman, but the philosophical essence of one of the foremost microbiologists in the world. Francis Krick was a winner of the Nobel Prize.

And thirty-some years later, here we are. Those responsible for the AIDS epidemic have at long last created the perfect tool for their Malthusian solution to their most pressing problem: Population control.

Who are those people?

"Code Word" is one of the highest security ratings for classified government documents. "Code Word Cardinal" is the password to the file containing intelligence information on a small group of the world's most powerful people. Some intelligence officers call them "Force X." They call themselves "The Olympians." They stand behind numerous organizations that deal in areas of global policy—such as the Global 2000 Committee and the Club of Rome—and even the closed and elite circle of government officials who know of their existence and some of their activities stand in awe at their power to dictate to governments and multinational corporations they control through ownership —or fear.

Their ruthlessness is well known to those who might fantasize about opposing them—or blowing the whistle on them. There's nowhere to hide. These families rule the world—and they take that power as their absolute, God-given right, and destroy without mercy anyone who might seriously threaten their privilege.

The existence of this group—let's call them "The Olympians," just as they call themselves—is one of the best-kept secrets of the 20th Century. And what they've done to mold life and humanity to their will—from the scourge of pellagra through the AIDS epidemic—is the scandal of the century. AIDS is merely their latest—and potentially most ruthless and destructive—form of warfare against ordinary humanity.

CHAPTER FOUR

This aristocratic tradition of "population control" found its expression in America in the early 20th Century with the formation in 1904 of what was then known as the "Station for Experimental Evolution." Funded by generous grants from Andrew Carnegie—who stated publicly that he was a hearty supporter of Malthus' ideas on "population control"—Cornelius Vanderbilt, J. P. Morgan and John D. Rockefeller, the Station conducted experiments involving different races.

One of their goals was to learn how to curb the rapid birth rate of blacks and other "coloreds." As outrageous as it may sound now, this was a goal that was very much on the minds of the Eastern rich in America. They were as frightened of being overrun by the masses—particularly the blacks—as the British had been of the natives they ruled in their colonies.

In 1910, Mrs. E. H. Harriman donated 80 acres of land at Cold Spring Harbor, Long Island, and $300,000 to the Station for Experimental Evolution to establish a "Eugenics Records Office." The widow of the man who created America's first great railroad fortune—the man who bankrolled the posse clever enough to track Butch Cassidy and the Sundance Kid, frightening them off to South America—her fortune was estimated at somewhere around a half billion dollars.

The newspapers called her the richest woman in the world, and she became a driving force behind eugenics research in America. (Eugenics is defined as "the study of hereditary improvement by genetic control.") The thrust of the research conducted at Cold Spring Harbor was to improve the superiority of the white race. Mrs. Harriman wanted a world-wide campaign of sterilization of defectives "to make race perfect." The creation of a Master Race, in other words.

The records of that era which are still available indicate that this was a socially acceptable view among the rich who supported Cold Spring Harbor. They were determinedly making plans to halt the birth rate of blacks and colored people—Indians and Asians—especially in Africa and the United States. A typical attitude among this group was expressed publicly by the vice president of the Immigration Restriction League, Madison Grant, a friend of Teddy Roosevelt's and a trustee of the Museum of Natural History:

"In Europe today, the amount of Nordic blood in each nation is a very fair measure of its strength in war and its standing in civilization. In the City of New York, and elsewhere in the United States there is a native American Aristocracy resting upon layer upon layer of immigrants of lower races . . . It has taken us 50 years to learn that speaking English, wearing good clothes and going to school and church does not transform a Negro into a white man . . . Americans will have a similar experience with the Polish Jew, whose dwarf stature, peculiar mentality and ruthless concentration on self-interests are being grafted upon the stock of the nation. Indiscriminate efforts to preserve babies among the lower classes often results in serious injury to the race."

Grant was a worthy heir to the spiritual tradition of Thomas Malthus—and he summarized nicely the world view of those who poured their money into the eugenics work of Cold Spring Harbor, both then and in the future. From 1915 until shortly before World War II, the Olympians opened the facilities at Cold Spring Harbor to many of Germany's leading genetic scientists. They conducted extensive research into the origins of various races and designed eugenics experiments to rid the world of the mentally retarded—who were called "undesirables" or "defectives." Cold Spring Harbor gained the reputation as the world's leader in eugenics research. The scions of the most respected American families, such as the Harrimans, funded these experiments—which continue until this day and led to the creation of the AIDS virus.

In the early days, they weren't even terribly secretive. There were seven superrich families who just accepted as their God-given privilege that they would someday own America—its natural resources and productive capacity—outright. Their ideas were not much advanced beyond feudalism. And they were so certain in their self-righteous rectitude that they openly told the press exactly what they planned. The press respectfully, even admiringly, published it. (Not completely unlike today's press.) These were the actual headlines from the New York World newspaper on September 4, 1915:

"Mrs. E. H. Harriman Backs a Gigantic Step in Eugenics Would Curb Defectives by the Hundreds of Thousands Over Series of Years.
To Make Race Perfect.
Aid of Rockefeller and Carnegie Hoped For in World-Wide Campaign."

The story began: "A world-wide campaign for the sterilization of defectives is called for in a report to the Eugenic Society, which has its headquarters at Cold Spring Harbor, Long Island and is generously aided financially by Mrs. E. H. Harriman. John D. Rockefeller and Andrew Carnegie are expected to contribute."

The Eugenics Office inflicted its cruelty from the beginning. Very early on, in 1915, they discovered in their scientific research that pellagra—a disease that still inflicted a high death toll—was caused by an insufficiency of niacin. The cure was a simple dietary one. Instead of spreading that information publicly, the Eugenics Office urged a diet of corn, which provides no niacin, and then viciously attacked other medical researchers who claimed that niacin prevented pellagra.

In particular, Mrs. Harriman ordered the Eugenics Office director, William Davenport, to heap contempt on the "niacin theory." She knew he wouldn't let her down. What had drawn her to hire him in the first place was an article in which he singled out the Irish as "defectives who genetically were not able to ward off tuberculosis." So with that moral and scientific view of humanity, he had no qualms about complying with her demand.

Financed by Mrs. Harriman, he published voluminous position papers discrediting the theory about niacin. Naturally, the Eugenics Records Office carried great weight in the medical community, and as a result, it was not until 1935 that the evidence about niacin was so incontrovertible that the Cold Spring Harbor theory—and its recommended corn diet—were discredited. But the fraud worked. During that generation, from 1915 to 1935, the Records Office stated that millions of "undesirable Southern poor whites and negroes died from the ravages of pellagra."

In 1932, the Third International Conference of Eugenics was held at the Museum of Natural History in New York City. It was sponsored by Mrs. H. R. duPont of the Delaware duPont family and a short roster of America's wealthiest—and most rabid—racists masquerading as environmentalists and eugenics benefactors: Mrs. Mary Averill Harriman, Major Leonard Darwin—the son of Charles Darwin, famous for his "Survival of the Fittest" natural selection philosophy—Mrs. John T. Pratt, Mrs. Walter Jennings, Dr. J. Harvey Kellogg, Henry Fairchild Osborn, Colonel William Draper and Mr. and Mrs. Cleveland H. Dodge.

Mrs. Pratt was of the Standard Oil Pratts, as was Mrs. Jennings. Kellogg made his fortune from breakfast cereal—and was widely known for the "eccentricity" of his views. Colonel Draper founded the Draper Foundation (which later used Robert Strange McNamara, Maxwell Taylor and McGeorge Bundy to forward its racial-environmental views) and Mr. Dodge was the financial brains behind President Woodrow Wilson, who rhapsodized lovingly about the environment in his 1913 inaugural address not long before he geared up to send American troops into the carnage of World War I.

These people wanted the natural resources of the world preserved for the present and future use of their own friends and families. They had no use whatsoever for the world's "useless eaters," as Lord Russell called them. In the modern vernacular, their views would be seen for what they were: unregenerately racist—pure and simple. It was no accident that the founders of the modern day environmentalist movement were the heirs to the great petroleum and pharmaceutical fortunes; they valued the resources of the planet more highly than ordinary human life. Those millions who were poor—or worse, poor and non-white—had no good reason to live.

The Conference unanimously elected Dr. Ernst Rudin as

president of the International Federation of Eugenics Organizations. Later, as co-author (with a member of the German Society for Racial Hygiene) of Hitler's law "For the Protection of German Blood and German Honour," Rudin earned himself a permanent niche in the pantheon of racism. (Hitler's law, incidentally, was based on a model developed at Cold Spring Harbor, the "Model Eugenical Sterilization Law" drafted in 1921.)

Henry Fairchild Osborn, a nephew of J. P. Morgan, was appointed vice president of the Conference. Osborn was the first known "racial-environmentalist" who connected "environmentalism" (a word invented by a close friend of Teddy Roosevelt) and "population control." Two years later, Osborn was awarded the Goethe medal by Hitler. In the light of the AIDS epidemic of the last 15 years, consider Osborn's opening speech to this august group in 1932:

"The outstanding generalization of my world tour are what may be summed up as 'six overs': overdestruction of natural resources, now actually worldwide, overmechanization in the substitution of the machine for animals and human labor, rapidly becoming worldwide, overconstruction of warehouses, ships, railroads, wharves and other means of transport, replacing primitive transportation; overproduction both of food and the mechanical wants of mankind, chiefly during the post-war (WWI) speculative period; overconfidence in future demand and supply, resulting in too rapid extension of both natural resources and mechanical equipment; overpopulation beyond the land areas or the capacity of the natural and scientific resources of the world, with consequent permanent unemployment of the least fitted.

"I have reached the opinion that overpopulation and underemployment are twin sisters. From this point of view I even find that the United States is overpopulated at the present time. In nature the less fitted individuals would gradually disappear, but in civilization, we are keeping them in the community in the hopes that in brighter days they may find employment. This is only another instance of humane civilization going directly against the order of nature and encouraging the survival of the unfittest."

In that same year, 1932, Cold Spring Harbor made its facilities available to German scientists working on racial concerns being voiced by Hitler and the burgeoning Nazi movement. In 1935, the Eugenics Records Office hosted a Conference on World Population in Berlin, and the American delegates included those already listed. The keynote speaker was German Interior Minister Wilhelm Frick. An American, Dr. Clarence G. Campbell, addressed the conference:

"The leader of the German nation, Adolf Hitler, ably supported by Dr. Frick and guided by Germany's anthropologists and social philosophers, has been able to construct a comprehensive policy of population development and improvement that promises to be epochal in racial history. It sets a pattern which other nations and other racial groups must follow if they do not wish to fall behind in racial quality, in their racial accomplishments and in their prospects for survival."

In the years immediately prior to World War II, the Harrimans' Cold Spring Harbor facilities remained open to Nazi Germany's leading genetic scientists, who then returned home and used their knowledge to forward Hitler's program of medical experiments designed to create a Master Race. From the documents I've been able to obtain, it is clear that the Eugenics Records Office pioneered racial experiments which were subsequently carried out in Nazi Germany—and may have been the model for Goering's T4 program, which, it is alleged, resulted in the killing of 400,000 mental patients who were classified as "defectives."

What we are seeing today, the AIDS epidemic, had its roots in the Cold Spring Harbor Eugenics Records Office, with its goal of curbing and reducing the birth rate of Negroes, Jews, "defectives" and "the layers upon layers of lower races." But, ultimately, Cold Spring Harbor scientists did more than show the way to a reduction in the birth rates of "undesirables." They succeeded in showing the way to murder millions of Lord Russell's "useless eaters."

CHAPTER FIVE

It's all happened very fast. Except in a few top secret, carefully guarded laboratories, AIDS did not exist in the United States before 1978—not in stored blood, not in humans, not anywhere. No American was infected with AIDS. In its first fifteen years, the virus has infected more than a million—perhaps two million—Americans, each of whom is infectious to others.

Although most of us remain unwilling to face the brutal facts, AIDS is the greatest crisis America faces—and perhaps ever has faced or ever will face. Future historians will write that mankind's greatest tragedy occurred while the leadership of the world's richest country either ignored what was happening—or contributed to the disaster. It's almost as if the great French author, Albert Camus, foreshadowed the future in his classic novel, *The Plague*, published in 1948:

"Small official notices had been put up about the town, though in places where they could not attract much attention. It was hard to find in these notices any indication that the authorities were facing the situation squarely. The measures enjoined were far from Draconian and one had the feeling that many concessions had been made to a desire not to alarm the public."

That desire not to alarm the public is best symbolized by the fact that the AIDS epidemic had begun its deadly course when Ronald Reagan was sworn in as president in 1981—and in his eight years in the White House, he barely uttered the word, or acknowledged the epidemic, in public. And the political climate of the era—and toward the disease—allowed him to get away with his complete abdication of leadership. If we had only the word of the American president to rely on, there was no AIDS epidemic during the Eighties.

As a result of the staggering head start the epidemic gained over any responsible public health authorities, here's where we stand today: AIDS has already killed more than twice as many Americans as died in the Vietnam war. Another million or two Americans are infected with the HIV virus—and facing a certain death sentence. In the greater New York-New Jersey area, according to an intelligence source, one in every four men visiting the twenty-six regional hospitals has tested positive for HIV. That's one-in-four ! In San Francisco, intelligence estimates are that half of the gay population would test positive.

AIDS is already the number one killer of black women of child-bearing age. As part of a research program on the likelihood of drastically slowing down the black population increases, the CIA predicted that Atlanta, with its large black population, would have 380,000 AIDS cases by 1992. The total number of AIDS cases in the U.S., the CIA estimated, would be 1.3 million, with roughly forty-six percent black, sixteen percent Hispanic, fourteen percent "other" races and the remainder white.

The same report said that a black woman is thirteen times more likely to get AIDS than a white woman, and Hispanic women are eleven times more likely. The CIA report stated: "Because of the high rate of infection among young black women and children, we see the black population growth being limited, and unless transmission (of the HIV virus) is interrupted, we may see zero population growth for blacks by the year 2010."

The federal agency responsible for controlling the outbreak of epidemics, the Centers for Disease Control in Atlanta, recently circulated a secret memo to its top officials estimating that one out of eight children born in America today will die of AIDS before they reach the age of 50.* A secret CIA report has concluded that twenty-five percent of Americans now showing symptoms of AIDS are in their early twenties—which means they contracted the disease while teenagers. "For every documented case of a young person testing positive for the HIV virus," the CIA report continues, "there are 1,000 others who carry the highly active virus, without even being aware of it."

Much of the rest of the world has suffered—and will suffer—an even worse fate. In Africa, the great AIDS plague rages out of

---

* The AIDS pandemic among infants infected by mothers is rapidly becoming one of the most pressing problems in our society.

The isolation of HIV retroviruses from cell-free breast milk has been noted in every instance where the mother has AIDS. Transmission of HIV through the acellur fraction of the milk has not been frequently noted. The American Medical Association does not, however, entirely exclude this possibility:

"The possibility that breast-fed infants acquired HIV infection from mothers via infected colostic leukocytes cannot really be excluded. This is because there are 1,000 to 2,000 x 10s/L viable macrophages normally contained in colostrum and human milk ingested by the neonate. Even though transfer of maternal cells through the infant gastrointestinal tract occurs, it would not be expected that the foreign cells could survive for a long time in the host, though it is likely the foreign cells can persist long enough to transmit HIV."

The idea that a nursing baby could only become infected by HIV viruses coming in direct contact with lesioned or broken mucous membranes has now been thoroughly discredited. It is now known that the retrovirus can enter the bloodstream through the skin without any open abrasions or ruptures of the skin being present.

control. Whole regions of Africa have been decimated; entire families and villages wiped out. The continent has one tenth of the world's population and sixty-four percent of reported AIDS cases.

In 1983, Jean Denezet, one of the French bankers who was present during McNamara's 1970 speech on population control, told *Le Figaro,* the newspaper most closely aligned with the French government: "World financial crisis will become virtually inevitable. Political consequences, just like in 1930, will be serious, but this time they will take place in the Third World."

Denezet made other remarks that *Le Figaro* chose not to publish. Here's the rest of what Denezet said in 1983: "Horrible things are going to happen in the Third World—and there is nothing to do, but just let it happen. Three and a half billion people are going to be plunged into a Hell worse than the Middle Ages." (Note the reference to the Middle Ages, with its oblique overtone of another Great Plague.)

Denezet knew what he was talking about. Since 1983, Africa has indeed been Hell worse than the Middle Ages. According to Dr. E. O. Idusogie, of the FAO regional office in Accra, Ghana, "about 100 million people in Africa are suffering from malnutrition (a euphemism for starving); AIDS carries away thousands every day, and civil wars in the region are causing chaos, confusion and a total breakdown of even the most meager sanitary conditions."

In 1989, Dr. Bernard Debre, a member of the French National Assembly, was interviewed by *Paris Match* upon his return from a tour of the continent. "Africa, engulfed by AIDS, is in a terrible situation because the disease thrives upon fragile populations; practically all (black) Africans are infected with malaria and parasites. . . . In Zaire, when we do blood tests, one out of four is contaminated with AIDS. All of the African countries are hit, and in some countries the disease reaches terrible proportions. Congo, Ivory Coast, Gabon, Cameroon, are severely hit. Zaire or Burundi may die." He estimated that perhaps thirty or forty percent of the populations were already infected with AIDS. "Poverty in Africa makes a serious fight against AIDS almost impossible."

While in the U.S., men with AIDS outnumber women with AIDS by seven to one, in Africa it is a family disaster. Women in Africa are more likely than men to die of AIDS. Four out of five AIDS sufferers in Zimbabwe are women. Among women in Africa, AIDS is spreading 100 times faster than it is in the U.S. According to an intelligence report, new, more virulent strains of the AIDS virus are surfacing. These have appeared in thousands of cases where persons tested showed false-negative results. It is believed that HIV testing simply did not identify the new strains.*

Brazil, with its large black population, has the highest incidence of AIDS in Latin America—second only to Africa. Brazil will see the deaths of millions from AIDS before the end of this decade. There will come a day sometime in the not-too-distant future when the toll from AIDS will be higher than all the deaths—about forty million—from all nations, in World War II.

---

* The normal AIDS test is called ELISA, which is followed by the Western Blot test, which is more expensive. (It measures the way the immune system reacts to each of the proteins contained in HIV viruses.) In Western Blot tests done in Africa, an increasing number of persons are showing a profile which is not complete, which would tend to be interpreted as indicating the presence of a newer, as yet, unidentified AIDS virus.

The same intelligence report says that the percentage of women contracting AIDS in African countries has shown a steep rise. The same holds true of children. "Thus we see a pattern arising which was not unexpected, but which nevertheless has caused some surprise by the swiftness in which the new HIV virus is now attacking women in African countries."

Lord Bertrand Russell's dream will have been realized by his spiritual heirs: the world's population will have been drastically thinned without all the wasteful munitions expense valuable property required by conventional warfare. AIDS is the ideal weapon of mass destruction.

Perhaps it was summarized best by Don Rowe, in his analysis for the *Wall Street Digest:* "The AIDS Plague will affect society in ways that you cannot now imagine. AIDS is 100 percent fatal. Scientists and medical research people are not optimistic about an immediate cure. They do not expect to develop an effective vaccine within the next two decades. Public Health officials estimate that 2.4 billion people (half the world's population) will die from AIDS within the next fifteen to twenty years. Economically, the insurance and medical health systems could be devastated in the 1990's. Nothing short of a spectacular medical breakthrough will keep Western civilization from suffering the worst catastrophe in the history of the world."

CHAPTER SIX

AIDS is the biogenetic equivalent of the atom bomb. The "Manhattan Project," the secret program to develop the bomb, had its beginnings in 1939 with a letter from Einstein to President Roosevelt alerting him that German physicists had recently entered an historically new realm in their research and would someday be capable of creating an explosive, based on the splitting of the atom, that would be unimaginably more destructive than any other weapon ever known to mankind. From that moment on, it was a certainty that the weapon would be built—and used—someday.

I don't know when the virus that would kill by destroying the human immune system was first conceived in some scientist's brain. But intelligence reports indicate that the actual laboratory experiments—at Fort Detrick, Los Alamos and Cold Spring Harbor—began during the 1960s.

How were the experiments conducted? According to intelligence documents, under the heading "Common Genetic Alterations of RNA," virologists mixed and cultured a combination of bovine leukemia virus and sheep maeda-visna virus. (Maeda-visna produces a nervous system degenerative disease in sheep, plus a lung infection, that is one hundred percent fatal. The entire sheep population of Iceland was wiped out by an epidemic between 1930 and 1950.)

These deadly animal viruses, on their own, could not leap the species barrier between animal and man. Bovine leukemia virus is deadly in cows, but not harmful to man; the same holds true of sheep maedi-visna virus. In all of nature, there were only a handful of known viruses—including Yellow Fever, Smallpox, Dengue Fever and Lassa Fever—capable of the leap between species.

But the bovine and sheep viruses were repeatedly injected into human tissue in the Fort Detrick labs until they actually mutated by incorporating human genes. Eventually the desired "cocktail mix" which humans could host was obtained. Once it was established that the virus could become a "natural" human infection, experiments proceeded with human body fluids, which were repeatedly injected with the successful "mix." The Fort Detrick virologists learned that the surest way to transfer the new "virus cocktail" to man was by repeated injections, such as occur when drug "partners" use the same needle, or through certain types of sexual activities frequently engaged in by homosexuals.

According to intelligence reports, the virologists at Fort Detrick drew heavily on the work of Russian scientists N. N. Vorobeva and G. D. Zaleski. They claimed that virally mutated vaccines artificially triggered many of today's diseases which were not common a hundred years ago. The Russians believed, for instance, that smallpox vaccines could cause hardening of the arteries. What the Fort Detrick researchers found was that herpes is the most important factor in the AIDS structure. The herpes virus, they wrote, activated the HIV virus to perform its deadly work.

This may sound like the script from a horror movie, but the fact remains that the virologists and scientists in the CAB labs did produce an unnatural creation—a new genetic "cocktail," half-animal, half-human, a certain killer capable of making the species leap.

Here is how Dr. Seale described their invention: "The AIDS virus (human immunodeficiency virus or HIV) is a lentivirus—a little-studied sub-family of the retroviruses. It is highly pathogenic to man, but it differs profoundly from any other virus of humans. It is the first virus to have appeared in mankind for many centuries which is entirely new, highly lethal and spreading steadily from person-to-person worldwide." (He added that retroviruses of animal origin, when repeatedly passed between human cells, would gain a preference for infecting human cells, perhaps even ceasing to be infectious to the animal hosts.)

This was not a well-meant endeavor that went haywire. This was not the work of a mad scientist. This was a project coldly calculated to discover whether a new virus could be created that would decimate a population in a seemingly "natural" plague. The experiments were concluded in 1967.

Thus was born the AIDS virus.*

* It is important to remember that there is absolutely no evidence of AIDS in Africa prior to 1967. There was one case, a British sailor who died of unknown causes in a hospital near Manchester, England, in 1958, that was very conveniently post-diagnosed many years later as AIDS. What really happened was this: When the experiments at Fort Detrick began, virologists at Porton Down in England recalled the incident with the sailor and sent tissues, which were preserved in paraffin, from the dead man's body to Fort Detrick for analysis.

Apparently the Fort Detrick virologists were able to establish that the sailor had died of one of the rare viruses capable of making the leap from animal to man. It could have been Lassa Fever. But intelligence reports indicate that this single sample was a great help to the virologists. Using technology that was not available when the sailor died in 1958, they retrieved DNA text sequences from his tissue, which provided them a vast amount of new information on retrovirus production.

* * *

The Chemical and Bacteriological Warfare labs were under heavy pressures to produce deadly new weapons. With the Vietnam War raging, relations between the two great superpowers had deteriorated to worse than ever. There was real paranoia in both governments about the other's intentions and capabilities. So in 1969, it came as a terrible shock for those in the know when British and U.S. intelligence discovered alarming evidence that a team of Soviet virologists, working under Victor Zhdanov —then the top virologist in the Soviet Union—had successfully isolated a retrovirus from human leukemia cells contaminated with "fetal calf serum." That put the Soviets ahead in this weapons race! It took a while longer for the Western labs to demonstrate how human leukemic cells could host the growth of bovine visna virus.

This would explain why veterinarians participated in the Fort Detrick "trials," and why the U.S. government subsequently gave Dr. O. W. Judd, a leading veterinarian, $8.5 million to study leukemia when human leukemia does not occur in animals. Why was a leukemia study conducted at a Harvard veterinarian college? Intelligence reports shed some light. Researchers at Fort Detrick were in possession of all of the documentation on the unsuccessful forty-year search for a vaccine to counter maedi-visna in sheep and eight-year search for a vaccine to counter infectious anemia in horses.

The experiments included infectious anemia of horses, a lentivirus and a cousin of leukemia in humans.* The tests were to

---

Then they used their delayed autopsy to further the cover story. They announced that this sailor had died of AIDS—in 1958.

*America's young middle class is being seriously damaged by AIDS-related diseases, the latest to emerge being Chronic Fatigue Syndrome. A

see whether the new "cocktail" could be carried to humans by horseflies (its normal methods of transmission; it is not a sexually transmitted disease in horses) and by other stinging insects. In frequency of infection and efficiency of "contact," the tests using human tissue were successful in establishing infection.

The significance of this lies in the fact that elements of all three viruses—horse and sheep and bovine—appear in humans infected with the AIDS virus. It is also significant that these are "retroviruses." When they penetrate a cell, they actually alter its genetic content. Which is exactly what happens when a person becomes infected with the HIV virus. The sheep maedi-visna retrovirus closely resembles the HIV virus. The bovine visna so closely resembles the HIV virus that it was actually called, at the time, BIV—bovine immunodeficiency-like virus.

The race was on. Congress was quietly notified on July 1, 1969 of the new biogenetic weaponry that was coming. A Department of Defense expert on biological warfare, Dr. McArthur, in testimony before the House Appropriations Committee actually described what we now know as the AIDS virus: "Within the next five-to-ten years," he said, "it probably will be

---

study by the Wister Institute revealed that the AIDS virus HTLV-II, a supposedly deadly "sleeper," is now being found in all reported cases of Chronic Fatigue Syndrome.

Many researchers believe that the HTLV-II (hairy cell leukemia virus) came into being after the Fort Detrick experiments. "Chronic Fatigue Syndrome" was a rarity a little more than ten years ago, but then during the late 1980s, a wave of HTLV-II hit the U.S., reaching frightening levels. Intelligence estimates are that a few million young Americans were infected. Did "Chronic Fatigue Syndrome" really just suddenly begin in the last few years? It almost certainly began ten years earlier, but went undetected. One intelligence report said "it might be as long as fourteen years before seroconversions show up in tests."

possible to make a new infective microorganism which would differ in certain important aspects from any known disease-causing organism. Most important of these is that it might be refractory to the immunological and therapeutic process upon which we depend to maintain our relative freedom from infectious disease. The total cost of such a program, which we could complete in five years, is in the region of $10 million."

He made these statements more than a decade before the first reported AIDS case in America!*

On October 2, 1970, former Secretary of Defense Robert S. McNamara—famous for his "body count" strategy in Vietnam —explained to a group of international bankers the dangerous situation they faced. "We can begin with the most critical problem of all," he said. "Population growth. It is the gravest issue that the world faces over the decades immediately head." At present trends, he announced, the world's population would not stabilize until about the year 2020—at a population of about ten billion, more than double the population of 1970.

---

* That something very strange—and dangerous—was going on did not escape the awareness of certain top scientists. Nobel laureate biochemist Joshua Lederburg warned of the dangers of monochlonal antibodies, which are protein antibodies that recognize and bind to foreign substances such as diseased cells, thus forming a critical element in our immune system. Married cells are called hybridomas. What Lederburg was concerned about was that the research at Fort Detrick involved antibody production in quantities previously not possible by natural means.

Why would that be worrisome to a Nobel laureate? Because the thrust of the Fort Detrick experiments with hybridomas was to find ways and means of defeating the human body's immune system; not to uncover ways and means of producing a greater supply of antibodies. This was how Fort Detrick virologists and neuropharmacology scientists discovered that neurotoxins carried in CAB weapons could be directed to attack the nervous system and the brain, inducing rapid loss of consciousness followed by an even more rapid onset of paralysis. Mixing such substances with HIV viruses became a daunting task, but it was successfully completed.

"We can assume that the levels of poverty, stress, hunger, crowding and frustration that such a situation could cause in the developing nations—which by then would contain nine out of ten human beings on earth—would be unlikely to assure social stability, or political stability. Or, for that matter, military stability."

Clearly, McNamara was letting the "haves" of the world know of the chaos they faced if they took no action. "It is not a world that any of us would want to live in," he said. "Is such a world inevitable? It is not sure, but there are two possible ways in which a world of ten billion people can be averted. Either the current birth rates must come down more quickly. Or the current death rates must go up. There is no other way.

"There are, of course, many ways in which the death rates can go up. In a thermonuclear age, we can accomplish it very quickly. Famine and disease are nature's ancient checks on population growth, and neither one has disappeared from the scene." One intelligence source informed me that McNamara was alluding to the development of new bacteriological warfare methods—and that he actually discussed them with certain carefully selected delegates after the conference.

McNamara was presumably speaking tongue-in-cheek about nuclear war. Not even Lord Russell would have advocated that solution. But as head of the World Bank and a former Defense Secretary and leading spokesman for Olympian causes, McNamara knew of the secret work being done with Chemical and Bacteriological Weapons. He knew that bacteriological weapons were feasible. He also knew about National Security Memorandum 200, authored by General Brent Scowcroft (who later became National Security Advisor to President Bush), which stated that U.S. political and economic interests "will require that the President and Secretary of State treat the subject of population growth control in the Third World as a matter of paramount importance."*

The research into this biogenetic form of population control was a carefully guarded secret. Nothing leaked into the news media—just as nothing leaked during the years when thousands of scientists and engineers and workers were creating a nuclear bomb in the "Manhattan Project." The only glimpses available even now come from old intelligence reports and esoteric scientific publications. One of the intelligence documents said that during 1972 the work at Cold Spring Harbor focused on the genetic control of immune responsiveness relative to a deadly new virus.†

But there were clues, even in the public record, if anyone had known where to look—and what they meant. In 1972, the World Health Organization—a witting participant—let an elite audience of scientists know that funding would be available to those who would pursue the creation of a hybrid virus that would be deadly to humans: "An attempt should be made to see

---

* The U.S. State Department has participated in many covert operations designed to thin the population of poor countries, notably in Cambodia, where the project was overseen by Thomas Enders, and in Nicaragua, by Thomas Ferguson, The State Department's case officer for the region.

† Many years later, in 1984, three courageous virologists, David Baltimore, Robert Weiss and Dr. Seale all expressed the belief that by the early 1970s, the laboratory techniques and technology to create new recombinant retroviruses of terrible virulence to mankind was already fully developed. All three men said that outside of laboratory testing, recombinations of retroviruses has never been known to occur naturally in humans.

The significant difference between the AIDS-HIV virus and any and all other recombinant retroviruses is that once in the human body, the cells of the infected person are genetically altered forever and the replication of the virus is astonishingly rapid. The AIDS victim now has a completely new set of genes and henceforth, his sole function for as long as he lives is to produce more of the virus. The infected person's body becomes, so to speak, a human HIV virus "factory."

if viruses can, in fact, exert selective effects on immune functions. The possibility should be looked into that the immune response to the virus itself may be impaired if the infecting virus damages more or less selectively the cell responding to the virus." (*World Health Bulletin*, 1972, 47, 257 and Fed Proc 1972 31:1087)

That same year, the World Health Organization actually alluded to its plans. "In relation to the immune response, a number of useful experimental approaches can be visualized," WHO reported in the *Federation Proceedings of the United States*. "This would be particularly informative in sibships." What that meant was that observing the effects of the new virus on brothers and sisters would provide useful information. (The African people, who were the first to receive the virus, were used like experimental animals in a laboratory, as were homosexuals after that.)

In 1972, the virus was ready for its first live experiments.

By 1974, the National Academy of Sciences was aware that something of great secrecy and extremely high importance was going on at Fort Detrick and the CAB labs—and the National Academy cooperated by recommending that members of its committee "voluntarily defer experiments linking animal viruses."

By 1978, the Olympians showed the enormity of their ambitions. National Security Council Memorandum 46—which became known among the few who were privy to it as the "King Alfred Plan"—discussed one possible solution to the black nationalist movement in the U.S.: stopping the growing birth rate among blacks in America by the year 2000, using several types of deadly viruses. This was actually written and circulated at the highest levels of government in 1978.

AIDS did not exist in the United States prior to 1978. Not in humans, not in stored blood; not anywhere—except in the laboratories. No American was infected with AIDS. All U.S. AIDS infection has occurred since the preparation of the "King Alfred" National Security Memorandum.

The "King Alfred Plan" revealed that the U.S. government had been collecting blood types of every nation on earth. These samples were given to virologists at Fort Detrick—among whom was a Mr. W. D. Lawton—and British virologists T. W. Burrows and R. C. Morris at Porton Downs in England (the most advanced Chemical and Bacteriological Warfare lab outside the former Soviet Academy of Science in Novisibirsk), who reported that blacks were more likely than whites to become infected with the virus. They would also have a shorter incubation period before showing symptoms and earlier death.

The British report found that people with a certain Gc 1 gene were predisposed to the HIV virus, while a Gc 2 gene offered some protection. As one intelligence report said, "Extensive research by the British team came up with the conclusion that blacks and mulattos have Gc 1 genes while whites have Gc 2 genes. This, the team said, meant that Africa and Brazil would be the most likely places in which the AIDS epidemic might start—and where it would flourish. This is believed to be the principle upon which the decision to infect Africa and Brazil with AIDS first was based. After that, they only had to find a means of delivering the AIDS virus to large numbers of people —and the World Health Organization found it."

The cover for the introduction of AIDS into Africa and Brazil —with its large black population—would be the World Health Organization's massive "humanitarian" campaign to "eradicate smallpox for once and for all." It was perfect. It even matched the surest way to pass the virus: injection.

The WHO smallpox vaccines would be contaminated with the AIDS virus. The dangerous viral agent chosen to contaminate the vaccines was SV-40, an idea which sprang from the results of a near disaster years earlier with contaminated Salk Polio Vaccine. Until 1962, SV-40—which caused cancer in animals—was contained in polio vaccine shots, and research work in the Soviet Union and Holland had concluded that the SV-40 virus was widespread in bovine serum, including fetal calf serum (BIV).

Fort Detrick virologists discovered that the loci of scores of genes related to the body's immune system are located on chromosome 14. They also found that SV-40 has a strong affinity for chromosome 14. The scientists reported that this was the link—the attack by SV-40 on chromosome 14—which caused polio, cancer, leukemia and immune suppression.*

---

* Even more diabolical was the reconfirmation that IgA antibodies are found in large quantities in the mucous membranes of the mouth and nose. This is the body's first line of defense against threatening invaders. This particular group differs from the circulating IgA antibodies, which are a single molecule. IgA in tissues was found to be more densely concentrated than single molecule IgA in blood.

What was the significance of this? It lay in the fact that foreign substances, such as those taken by mouth, would more readily be overcome by the IgA antibodies in the mucous membranes of the mouth, than foreign substances introduced directly into the blood stream. Thus, injected vaccines were found to be "much better." Better for what? For helping a sick person recover or further weakening the immune system? There has been, for instance, a proliferation of cancer among those who received injections of smallpox vaccine—and as a direct result.

The Fort Detrick team observed another important factor: that age played a big role in determining how quickly injected foreign substances would react unfavorably. It was discovered that in experiments with lab mice, the old mice became convulsed and died very quickly when injected with vaccines, but the very young mice hardly reacted at all. What is frightening about this is that while the young mice did not die, they retained the inoculated viruses in their bodies all of their lives, most of them eventually succumbing to kidney failure.

The story of SV-40 first appeared publicly in "Human Exposures to SV-40: A Review and Comment," an article by noted epidemiologists N. Nathanson and K. Shah, published in the *American Journal of Epidemiology*. (Vol 103, No.1, January, 1976.) The article said that in the 1950s, millions of Americans were exposed to the papova virus SV-40, a common and unrecognized contaminant which had been prepared from virus pools grown in simian monkey kidney cultures. In February 1977, in "Science That Frightens Scientists," published in the *Atlantic Monthly*, William Bennett and Joel Gurin confirmed that millions of people in the U.S. were "inadvertently" injected with simian virus 40.

Subsequently it was confirmed that the Salk polio vaccine was cultured in kidneys from African green monkeys. This may have given rise to the myth that a man bitten by a green monkey contracted AIDS, which then developed into the present AIDS epidemic. As preposterous as it is, this fable is still one of the most accepted theories about the genesis of AIDS.

Given what we now know about the powerful contaminant SV-40, it was a miracle that the polio inoculation program wasn't a giant disaster. Many so-called "flu shots" during the presidency of Gerald Ford also contained SV-40, which may account for the fact that over twenty percent of those who received the shots became seriously ill and many died. In 1977 the government denied that SV-40 contamination of vaccines was deliberate.

The preponderance of evidence suggests that the government was—and still is—lying. Even as late as 1992, it was not known whether SV-40 is searched for in AIDS victims. The terrible danger here is that according to intelligence documents, SV-40 can lie dormant and then be "reactivated" or "triggered" when needed, which can also happen with HIV and two or three AIDS-related complex viruses.

In fact it has been demonstrated that SV-40 is one of the activators of HIV-AIDS viruses. This is confirmed in an article by Howard E. Gendelman, published in the *Proceedings of the National Academy of the United States of America*, vol. 83. Gendelman wrote that SV-40 can nullify the immune system, leaving the body open for attacks by other viruses.

Shortly after the World Health Organization's smallpox vaccination program was completed, serious outbreaks of AIDS occurred in Central Africa and Brazil. As early as 1984, several intelligence services—ranging from U.S. allies such as French intelligence and the Vatican to enemies such as the KGB and Libyan intelligence (which had access to sensitive information from the then highly efficient Rumanian intelligence service)—began circulating internal reports that the U.S. was running experiments with contaminated vaccines in human inoculations.

In 1985 The World Health Organization sent one if its top officials to soothe the anxiety of African governments whose people were suffering a wildfire of AIDS infection. He was supposed to deliver the official WHO message: AIDS was "no problem." But once the WHO official saw the situation first hand, he refused. But WHO continued to insist that the problem of AIDS in Africa was being grossly exaggerated.

About the same time, rumors began circulating that the AIDS epidemic in Africa had been spread by WHO's smallpox vaccinations. But evidence was hard to come by. The World Health Organization and other AIDS "authorities" simply dismissed the rumors as lunatic nonsense. Then, on May 11, 1987, Pearce

Wright, the Science Editor of the *London Times*, took the story public.

He wrote that he had been approached by a consultant formerly employed by the World Health Organization to do research into the smallpox vaccinations. Some officials—who were obviously unwitting—had become suspicious that the smallpox vaccine used by WHO in Africa was indeed infected with the AIDS virus. When the consultant finished his investigation and reported to WHO that the suspicions were correct—the vaccine was contaminated—WHO buried his report and sent him on his way.

After he did his own investigation, Wright reported: "WHO is studying new scientific evidence suggesting that immunization with the smallpox vaccine awakened unsuspected, dormant HIV infection. Some experts fear that in obliterating one disease, another disease was transformed from a minor endemic illness of the Third World into the current pandemic (of AIDS). A WHO advisor who disclosed the problem told *The Times*, 'I believe the smallpox vaccine theory is the explanation to the explosion of AIDS . . . It would account for the position of each of the seven central African states which top the league table of the most affected countries; why Brazil became the most afflicted Latin American country; and how Haiti became the route for the spread of AIDS to the U.S. It also provides an explanation of how the infection was spread more evenly between males and females in Africa than in the West and why there is less sign of infection among five to 11-year-olds in Central Africa. The greatest spread of HIV infection coincides with the most intense immunization program.' "

Jon Rapport, writing in *Easy Rider* on June 4, 1987, confirmed Wright's story and added what he had learned in Washington: "Contaminated vaccines made in tissue cultures of animal parts contain 'extra dangerous viruses' and WHO smallpox vaccine doses may have been contaminated in this fashion. According to investigations carried out by a team of doctors from the Walter Reed Hospital, there is a definite connection between vaccines and AIDS."

Evidence for that connection had actually been in the public record since 1969—in the early stages of the AIDS project. During a workshop at the National Institutes of Health at Bethesda, Maryland on July 27-30, and partly sponsored by the World Health Organization, Dr. D. B. Amos presented a paper in which he stated: "In relation to the immune response, a number of useful experimental approaches can be visualized. One would be a study of the relationship of HL-A type to the immune response, both humoral and cellular, to well-defined bacteria and antigens, during preventative vaccinations. "

Since this paper was delivered several years prior to the outbreak of AIDS—at a time when no one had died from the disease—it seems safe to conclude that these mentions of "the HL-A type" and "the immune response" and "preventive vaccinations" were not made in pursuit of a cure.

CHAPTER SEVEN

Haiti was targeted next. But the Haitian experiment was not racial; it was aimed at homosexuals.

There has been great speculation about whether or not the AIDS virus originated in Haiti and was then brought into the United States by gay men who were infected there. This is an interesting concept worthy of special study. The abject poverty and crowding in insanitary slum areas in Haiti is well known. In the slums, it is almost impossible to tell one hut from another; a stream of water running through the middle of the quarter is filled with fecal matter, but that does not stop inhabitants from drinking it and using it to wash themselves. Family sanitation consists of a chamber pot passed around until it is filled, emptied outside and then reused before retiring to bed. It is not surprising that Haiti was a place waiting for an outbreak of the AIDS Plague.

But until the AIDS scare, Haiti was a very popular vacation spot for American gays. Carrefour in the center of Port-au-Prince has massive walls around it to keep out the fetid stench, sights and sounds of the slums. In Carrefour, anything goes. Any imaginable sexual desire could be gratified, at an affordable price. (Was this why AIDS became rampant in Haiti, but hardly occurred in its neighbor, the Dominican Republic?)

The "Haitian Connection" was uncovered quite by accident during a routine autopsy conducted on the body of a black male at Jackson Memorial Hospital in Miami. Although not known at the time of the autopsy, the dead man had come from Haiti. The victim was diagnosed as having succumbed to toxoplasmosis after the autopsy doctor saw that the Haitian's brain was speckled with blue spots, instead of being the normal strong pink color.

Then, an article in the *New York Times* in July, 1982, disclosed that thirty-two Haitian men living in Florida and New York were found to have rare diseases—toxoplasmosis, cytomegalovirus, Kaposi's sarcoma and pneumocystis—known to be "associated" with this new fatal illness that was striking down gays. During 1982, there were persistent stories in the news media and several so-called "alternative press" journals that Haiti had something to do with AIDS. Some went so far as to link AIDS in Haiti with zombies, but few—except among ardent believers in voodoo—gave that idea any credence.

In some voodoo ceremonies, the males present resort to buggery with pigs. Is this how African swine fever viruses were passed to humans? There is a great deal of medical evidence suggesting that swine fever closely parallels AIDS. For example, the fever suppresses the immune system of pigs and is thought to do the same in humans.

Dr. C. Prakash of the Ohio State Agricultural Research and Development Center said that certain male pigs are homosexual, and that they tend to get swine fever more easily than those who show no such tendencies. Apart from fever, other symptoms are pneumonia and a type of Kaposi's sarcoma. Dr. Prakash said that the African swine fever virus is found in urine, blood and semen of pigs, in much the same way as the AIDS virus is found in these fluids in humans.

Even more compelling was the fact that severe outbreaks of swine fever in parts of Africa, especially in Zaire, which has strong trade relations with Haiti, coincided with the serious outbreak of AIDS. A former Harvard School of Public Health scientist, Dr. Jane Teas, wrote several papers linking African swine fever to AIDS, and won public recognition from the Pennsylvania House of Representatives for her work in this area.

Intelligence documents show that in 1971 anti-Castro exiled Cuban leaders were given a vial of African swine fever which was then smuggled into Cuba and released among pigs. In 1977, the *Boston Globe* broke the news of this covert operation and said it was carried out "with at least the tacit approval of the U.S. Central Intelligence Agency." *Newsday* reported that an intelligence source had told them that the Cuban "was given the virus in a sealed, unmarked container at Fort Gutlick in Panama—a CIA training ground—with instructions to turn it over to the anti-Castro group."

Chuck Ortleb, publisher of the *New York Native* is one of many who believe that AIDS is the human version of African swine fever. With an outbreak of swine fever in the West—particularly in the U.S.—in 1971, shortly after the development of the AIDS virus, it seems legitimate to ask: Was the U.S. outbreak engineered to provide the cover for an attempted mass inoculation against swine fever? The government later abandoned the inoculation program, because of the outcry over the number of deaths it caused, particularly among the elderly.

Ortleb maintained that the introduction of swine fever virus into Haiti was probably deliberate, because it was well-known that many gays vacationed or stopped off in Port-au-Prince. "The parallels between the two diseases are overwhelming," he wrote. "I think gay people have got to see themselves as being murdered."

I agree. But while the swine-fever-AIDS virus was found in Haiti, it did not originate in that country. It was planted there after being "cocktailed" in laboratories at Cold Spring Harbor and Fort Detrick. Could the U.S. government really take part in such monstrous behavior? Don't ever forget Project MK-Ultra, in which thousands of unsuspecting people were dosed with LSD—with deadly consequences for some. If it weren't for the explosive pressures arising from the Watergate scandal, MK-Ultra would remain a secret to this day.

After the CIA experiment in Haiti, small numbers of AIDS cases began to be reported among homosexuals who had vacationed on the island. The first recorded case of this new disease in America was in March 1980. "Nick," a young gay man living on Fire Island, New York, went to see his doctor and complained of a strange illness. The symptoms "Nick" experienced were fever, loss of weight, extreme fatigue, swollen lymph nodes, bluish bumps over his body and diarrhea.

When "Nick" died, the autopsy report said he had succumbed to Toxoplasma gondii, a parasitic disease that invades the body cells. The parasites multiply rapidly, stretching cell walls until they break, sending hordes of parasites to invade new cells. The symptoms shown by "Nick" and the autopsy report confirmed that whatever he suffered from quite closely resembled Black Plague.

Among the diseases searched for by the autopsy were those common to gays with many sex partners: urethritis, shigella, amebiasis, scabies, hepatitis, syphilis, gonorrhea. None of these were found in "Nick's" body. Nor was there any trace of lymphogranuloma vencerum, a tropical disease found among homosexuals who had traveled to Haiti and Africa.

After "Nick's" death, reports began appearing in the American press about this strange new disease. On May 11, 1982, the *New York Times* carried a major story about a "new homosexual disorder," which it called "Gay Related Immunodeficiency" (GRID). (The disease was later given the name AIDS by Don Armstrong, chief of infectious diseases at the Memorial Sloane Kettering Cancer Center in New York, and first officially used in the Morbidity and Mortality Weekly Report published in the fall of 1982 by the Centers for Disease Control.)

But then came a sudden explosion of AIDS cases. The Haitian connection could not come close to squaring up with the big numbers being reported. The answer to how that could happen was known only to a few. While Fort Detrick had researched animal-human viruses, the Los Alamos lab in New Mexico had been given the task of finding out just how much faster the animal-RNA virus mutated in relation to human (natural) viruses. An intelligence report on the Los Alamos findings was written and then destroyed—but not before one copy was secreted out.

The results: In the first test, using two natural (DNA) viruses, placed side by side in the lab alongside an RNA-infected virus, replication difference in time amounted to less than 1.5 percent at the end of a year between the two natural viruses, or a total difference of under three percent annually. The infected RNA-virus mutated an astonishing 1 million times faster than the two DNA viruses.

The first case was reported in Uganda in 1972, so at the normal rate of replication it would have taken fifteen years to approach 8,000 cases. The doubling time for the numbers of people infected every 14 months in relation to the first reported cases in Africa and Brazil and Haiti proved beyond any reasonable doubt that a very substantial number of people had to have become infected with the AIDS virus, all more or less at the same time.

What really happened? Were homosexuals deliberately targeted for AIDS experiments?

Consider this: In 1969, a certain Dr. W. Szmuness was admitted to the U.S. by the Immigration and Naturalization Service. A Polish citizen, he was educated in the Soviet Union and had been serving as an advisor to the World Health Organization in Poland. British intelligence suspected him of being a KGB agent. And yet, he was admitted to the U.S. and immediately given the top job at the New York City Blood Bank. Why? In 1969, suspected KGB agents were not routinely welcomed into America and given high-level scientific jobs. The Justice Department would know the answer to that question, but they decline comment on Dr. Szmuness.

Once installed at the Blood Bank, Dr. Szmuness set up a major study of a Hepatitis B vaccine.* But here's the weird part: only sexually active male homosexuals between the ages of twenty and forty were allowed to participate. There was certainly no valid reason why a legitimate vaccine test should be limited to promiscuous young homosexuals. And yet it was. And the introduction of the hepatitis vaccine exhibited the exact symptoms and epidemiology of AIDS. Even chronic intestinal lymphoid pneumonia began appearing in the homosexuals who participated in the Hepatitis B study.

When the AIDS epidemic first appeared, the Centers for

---

* He also began an experimental program with the herpes virus. Some intelligence operatives believe this was meant to advance the Fort Detrick research on the role of herpes in "transactivating" the AIDS virus.

Disease Control claimed that only four percent of those in Dr. Szmuness' program had contracted AIDS. Four years later, the CDC admitted that the number was sixty percent. And then the CDC stopped giving numbers. Why? Because, intelligence sources told me, the number had reached one-hundred percent. Every single man who received Dr. Szmuness' Hepatitis B vaccine contracted the AIDS virus. Intelligence sources have confirmed that Dr. Szmuness' Hepatitis B vaccine was deliberately contaminated with the HIV virus to introduce AIDS massively and exclusively into the homosexual community in America's largest city.

CHAPTER EIGHT

The official version of how AIDS began is not well known—or documented. So it is perhaps worth an overview of how this disaster is supposed to have happened.

The prevalent cover story for the spread of the AIDS epidemic is that the source of the virus was the African green monkey. To this day, most people believe that AIDS began with infected monkeys biting people. But it would have taken hundreds of monkeys biting hundreds of people for the epidemic to have broken out in such massive numbers at virtually the same time and continents apart. If the MGM (mythical green monkey) story were true, there might be 20,000—or extravagantly, perhaps 50,000, or maybe even 100,000—cases in Africa, rather than the thirty million known cases by 1992.

The MGM story cannot withstand any serious scrutiny. Let us reject that theory out of hand. An exhaustive examination of a colony of green monkeys later revealed no trace of the AIDS virus. The AIDS virus does not occur naturally in the green monkey. According to intelligence information, the HIV virus had previously never occurred in any animals. And it has since been proven that it is genetically impossible to transfer any virus from green monkey cells to man. Not to mention that green monkeys don't exist in Brazil and Haiti.

Where did the MGM story come from? Perhaps from the fact that polio vaccines were cultured on green monkey kidney cells in the 1960s to produce the Salk polio vaccine. But the process went wrong and millions of people were injected with contaminated vaccine containing SV-40.*

Despite the desire to squash the underground rumblings around the world that AIDS is a creation of man, no government, including the U.S. government, has to date offered any persuasive theory—or evidence to back it—to support the belief that the AIDS epidemic sprang from nature and spread in the fashion it has. Simple logic should tell us this much: If nature was responsible for the AIDS virus and its catastrophic impact, don't you think that the U.S. government—with its massive intelligence-gathering apparatus, its nearly limitless scientific facilities and its access to the media—would by now know at least some of the answers and present a persuasive case?

Well, it hasn't. Not even close. Could anyone who reads this even answer the question: What does the U.S. government say caused AIDS? A lame theory about the African green monkey is the best they can do—and they haven't staked their credibility even on that. It's a question the government would prefer not to answer. Why not? Because they know that no matter what theory they put forth, it's not true—and there are too many scien-

---

* Many of those injected with the contaminated vaccine are today paying the price in an increase in the rates of cancer, multiple sclerosis and who knows what other diseases.

Multiple sclerosis, once a rare disease, spread like wildfire after the polio vaccine inoculation campaign. Although no specific records can be cited, some researchers believe that an increase in cancers can be traced to the introduction of contaminated vaccines.

tists around the world who would be able to discredit it. So they remain silent and trust that most people will not take the trouble to wonder why.

The federal bureaucracy officially responsible for protecting us from epidemics, the Centers for Disease Control in Atlanta, and its staunch ally in the dissemination of disinformation, *The Journal of the American Medical Association* (JAMA) have glossed right over the genesis of AIDS. Explaining the spread of a disease is quite different than explaining its origin. The CDC and JAMA stayed clear of that treacherous arena. Instead they chose to imply—and falsely—that AIDS is a sexual disease transmitted primarily by heterosexuals in Africa and homosexuals in the West.

The AIDS epidemic began with a mass movement of the population from the country to the cities in Africa, we are told, with a natural increase in sexual activity. "The urbanization of Africa has been accompanied by an increase in heterosexual activity and hyperendemicity gonorrhea," JAMA reported on October 24, 1985, by way of explaining the outbreak of AIDS.

"Aids was then transmitted on a global scale primarily through homosexually mediated behavior as underscored by virtually every epidemiological study available," reported JAMA. "In America this is reflected by 13:1 preponderance of infection in males as opposed to females, an 11:1 ratio in Europe and 26:1 ratio in Australia. Sixty to a hundred percent of the total number of cases in 12 of 16 countries in Europe are in homosexual men. Overall in Europe, 78 percent of cases are in homosexual/bisexual men, and homosexual transmissions combined with IV drug abuse accounts for 87% of European cases, with considerable overlap between the two groups here and in other countries.

"In Canada the vast majority of AIDS cases have occurred in homosexual-bisexual men living in the largest urban areas. Brazil has accounted for the second highest international toll of reported AIDS cases, far and away the highest per capita incidence in Latin America. Sao Paulo and Rio de Janeiro are two of the few places where homosexuality is tolerated and practiced openly, with the immediate result that Brazil's reported AIDS cases are concentrated in the large gay communities of these two cities."

In a report dated October 16, 1986, Drs. Curran and Mason of the Centers for Disease Control stated that three in thirty homosexual males between the ages of twenty and fifty were infected with the AIDS virus: "In California, New Jersey, Texas and Florida, the figure was 1 in 9 homosexual males between the ages of 30 and 39. Homosexual transmission accounts for 78 percent of U.S. cases, but this figure increases to 93 percent when combined with drug abusers."

Homosexual promiscuity—and the unique susceptibility of certain homosexual activities—and the gravely unsanitary conditions and urban crowding in African cities were undoubtedly factors in the spread of the virus. But that does not account for the massive outbreaks that occurred in rural tribal areas, which in Kenya, Uganda and Zaire, wiped out the population—all age groups—of whole villages and towns, where there was much less crowding and sanitary conditions were better. The AIDS virus in Africa was not caused by increased heterosexual activity; the very idea is preposterous. Why would an increase in heterosexual activity spread an epidemic that was confined to homosexuals and drug abusers in Western countries?

But their scapegoat strategy worked. A portrayal emerged in which the blame for AIDS was laid squarely upon African heterosexuals who moved to the city and drug abusers and gay communities in the West. Gays became the whipping boy of the world. This was intended to reassure the general population that if one were not homosexual or an intravenous drug abuser, there was no need to fear infection with the AIDS virus.

The media bought the story and passed it on to the public. Witness this account in the *Los Angeles Times* on August 8, 1987: "In the urban areas of the United States, Canada, Western Europe, Australia, Brazil and Mexico, the AIDS virus is usually transmitted through male homosexual contact (or to a considerably lesser degree) by intravenous drug users who share contaminated needles and syringes. There is relatively little heterosexual transmission of AIDS virus in these countries."

Totally missing from the CDC and JAMA conclusions is the answer to the most important question: Where had the AIDS virus come from ? Just try to get that answer from them. Like the curate's egg, parts of the CDC information are good, but parts are very bad. Take the reference to Brazil. Certainly Sao Paulo and Rio de Janeiro have a large gay presence, but to imply, as CDC did, that gays in these two cities caused an epidemic of AIDS to sweep Brazil to its furthest corners—even remote villages along the Amazon—defies logic and common sense. What those remote villages in Brazil and Africa shared in common was not a hedonistic gay lifestyle; what they shared in common was that they'd all been vaccinated against smallpox by the World Health Organization.

Here's the truth about the spread of the AIDS epidemic: Following successful experiments conducted against Zaire, AIDS was deliberately introduced into Africa. Because it has the largest black population outside Africa, Brazil was then targeted. Then came the Haitian connection—to begin the destruction of the homosexual community in America.

CHAPTER NINE

The destruction of the homosexual community has created one of the most dangerous myths we face about AIDS: that it is primarily transmitted by sexual contact. AIDS is not an "ordinary" venereal disease; a sort of deadly gonorrhea. AIDS is a blood-borne virus. As Dr. Daniel Benson of UCLA says, "blood is the major avenue of contamination."

That simple fact invalidates everything we've been taught to believe about the spread of AIDS. As Dr. John Seale explains: "Scientists and doctors have repeatedly stated as fact that the AIDS virus is fundamentally transmitted during sexual intercourse, but is, unfortunately, sometimes transmitted in blood. This is highly misleading, though published laboratory and epidemiological evidence, and editorials in scientific and medical journals, have been heavily slanted to support this "fact."

"In reality, AIDS is a characteristically blood transmitted infection, which is only transmitted with difficulty during sexual intercourse compared with the genuine sexually transmitted diseases gonorrhea and trichomonosias. All the exceptional epidemiological evidence is consistent with this view. Obviously AIDS is transmittable during sexual intercourse, but so is influenza, glandular fever and scabies. Sexual intercourse is only one of many ways by which the virus can be transmitted, and is by no means the most efficient . . .

"Having assumed for a variety of motives that AIDS is a sexually transmitted disease like syphilus or gonorrhea, a negligible research effort has gone into the critical matter of transmission. . . . As far as it goes, the tiny research effort into infectivity of bodily fluids indicates that saliva is far more infectious than genital secretions, but that blood and serum is vastly more infectious than either. Consequently the idea that condoms can have any significant effect on the spread of AIDS in a nation is utterly preposterous. Governments all over the world are spending millions of pounds advising their citizens to prevent AIDS by using condoms on the basis of manifestly fraudulent misrepresentation of scientific evidence presented by scientists themselves."

No lifestyle is safe enough to guarantee protection from infection. The terrible truth is that the risk for most people—who feel safe from the AIDS plague, because they are heterosexual, monogamous, drug-free—is far greater than is generally known. Dr. Seale: "People with AIDS are categorized as belonging to a small number of 'risk groups,' giving the false impression that the vast majority of people cannot get AIDS. AIDS is portrayed as only a behavioral disease caused by sexual and narcotic misdemeanors. This implies that if anybody gets AIDS, it is their own fault. Emphasis on transmission of the virus during sexual intercourse and education as a solution to the epidemic implies that the disease will disappear with modified behavior. This misses the point that as the epidemic explodes, infection by chance, non-sexual, contact becomes even more common."

How many Americans believe that even kissing can spread the virus? Here is what Dr. Marcello Piazza, a world renowned authority on AIDS, published in the *Journal of The American Medical Society* on January 13, 1989: "It is generally accepted that the presence of blood in saliva is indirect evidence that microlesions are present in the oral cavity. During kissing, two mucosae, both of which may contain microlesions come into close contact. The intense rubbing that occurs during kissing can favor both the creation of microlesions and the passage of blood from one partner to the other. If the blood of one partner contains HIV, the virus can pass into the bloodstream of the other partner.

"Our study has shown that microlesions are normally present in the oral mucosae and that saliva contains blood. Therefore, we feel that passionate kissing cannot be considered 'protective sex' for the transmission of human immunodeficiency virus infection. We found that blood is present in the saliva of fifty percent of subjects examined, its level increasing significantly after brushing of teeth or passionate kissing."

Two teenagers necking are at risk.

In a meeting in Montreal in 1989, several virologists and doctors confirmed that kissing will transmit AIDS. But government doctors and scientists who wanted to attend were told they would face "disciplinary action." So the meeting was boycotted by many who most needed to be present. But if kissing can pass the infection, how much value do condoms really have? Not much, if any.

"Safe sex" is a myth, knowingly created by our leaders to avoid public panic—or wrath. "Safe sex" is advertised as a panacea for AIDS. Big name stars are used to promote this deadly fraud. But condoms are not a solution for AIDS; they merely spread permissiveness—and put even more people in jeopardy, believing they are "safe" if they use them.

Dr. William O'connor, a noted AIDS researcher, has stated flatly: "Nearly every fluid in the human body is capable of transmitting the virus, including blood, saliva, tears and sweat. People have become infected by simply touching the blood of virus carriers or having microscopic quantities of infected blood strike their faces. Viruses have been cultured from the air of operating rooms. All that is required (to become infected) is that a single virus particle has to come in contact with a susceptible human cell."

One drop of infected blood is all it takes. Even now, in 1994, our blood supply is significantly more dangerous than Americans realize. The average American is under the impression that AIDS-contaminated blood was a problem a few years ago, but that it has been corrected and the supply is now completely safe. It is potentially a fatal mistake to believe that. Transfusion, in fact, still carries more risk of AIDS infection than the authorities want you to know.

Already, tens of thousands of Americans have contracted AIDS through blood transfusions—and that number grows daily. Take the terrible plight of American hemophiliacs. As long ago as March 1990, the *Journal of the American Medical Association* admitted that as many as sixty to eighty percent of America's hemophiliacs had been infected with AIDS through contaminated blood transfusions.

In spite of attempts by hospitals to limit their liability for administering transfusions of HIV-tainted blood, the next few years will see a flood of lawsuits by unknowing recipients. All Kaiser hospitals in San Francisco have been warned of this, and Kaiser admitted privately a few years ago that it believed they had already transfused an estimated 30,000 patients with HIV-tainted blood. But the American Red Cross continues to sell HIV-tainted blood to blood banks across the country.

Why the Red Cross? Doesn't the Red Cross do marvelous humanitarian work? Yes, it does, but in its management of blood banks, it has been criminally negligent. By allowing its computer management control of blood supplies to break down, the Red Cross was unable to properly monitor blood collected from donors. Passwords for computer entry were stolen and used to falsify computer records to cover up that blood allegedly tested had not been tested. The result was that thousands of people received HIV-contaminated blood. This showed up very quickly in hemophiliacs; over 2000 of them became infected by Red Cross blood. The Red Cross was forced to appoint an internal panel to sort out the mess it had made.

The Red Cross still hasn't instituted a uniform system of screening dangerous would-be donors, such as persons suffering from AIDS, Hepatitis or TB—even drug users who inject their poison. Dr. Robert Mendleson, a noted author, stated on a radio talk show that eighty percent of doctors surveyed would not accept Red Cross blood for use on themselves or their families.

Even as mainstream a magazine as *Money*, as recently as its May 1994 issue, carried a major expose, "America's Dangerous Blood Supply," detailing how AIDS carriers are still being allowed to donate blood. "After 10 years of testing donor blood for HIV," *Money* wrote in its ads for that issue, "Americans are still contracting the disease through transfusions. Remarkable as that may sound, what's even more startling is that these tragedies occur due to human error, flawed testing and legal loopholes. Not to mention the fact that the FDA, heavily influenced by the American Red Cross and other blood bank leaders, resisted adopting a more accurate blood test because it cost an additional $3. Why do concerns for cost outweigh those for human life?"

The answer is this: Blood is big business. American Red Cross blood revenues are approaching $100 million a year—much of it clear profit. The International Red Cross is a major trader in blood, receiving more than $4 billion a year in revenues around the world.

The problem may be even worse overseas. Poor countries without adequate facilities of their own are large markets for imported blood. One intelligence report monitoring infected blood supplied to targeted countries (India in this case) indicated that one million Indians have AIDS—twice as many as reported by the World Health Organization. Contaminated blood supplied to India contained HIV-1, HIV-II and HTLV-1 and HTLV-II.

Hospitals are the most vulnerable to a blood-borne virus. The one institution designed as a safe place to cure us of our ills is now on the front lines of spreading the infection. The number of hospital care workers with reported cases of AIDS rose from 1.7 percent in 1983 to 5.7 percent in 1987. And while assuring hospital care workers that they were not in a high risk category, the Centers for Disease Control recommended that they handle all patients as if they were infected with AIDS.

Have you visited a hospital recently and noticed the small, inconspicuous signs in bathrooms and hallways—under the headline "Universal Precautions"—reminding the staff to regard every patient as a potential carrier of blood-borne pathogens? They're sort of like the notices in Camus' *The Plague*: "One had the feeling that many concessions had been made to a desire not to alarm the public."

The small notices are a subtle way of reminding doctors and nurses and staff that everyone they encounter is a deadly threat. Even the tiniest mistake—say, an accidental prick of their skin from a used syringe—can now cost them their lives. Doctors and health care workers are instructed to wear masks, gloves and gowns—and not to give mouth-to-mouth resuscitation, using resuscitation bags instead. All wards must have such bags on hand.

"There is a growing sense of anxiety among American surgeons concerning the AIDS epidemic," says one intelligence agent, "and the high risk that all operating room personnel now face because of the heavy incidence of AIDS." AIDS is being spread in operating rooms through the use of high-speed power tools used as surgical instruments. Tests have now determined that the AIDS virus can live on dry surfaces outside the body for seven days and wet surfaces for fourteen days.

The Pasteur Institute has confirmed findings of live AIDS viruses on wet and dry surfaces outside the body, a stunning piece of news that the media managed to ignore. Stated the report: "Infectious virus was still detected after fifteen days at room temperature. Infectious virus could be recovered from dried material after up to three days at room temperature and in an aqueous environment survived longer than fifteen days."

Stanford University conducted tests for the U.S. Biological Warfare Department of the Department of Defense which showed that AIDS-contaminated blood deposited onto a surgeon's rotating drill contaminated the air with a fine aerosol mist, containing live HIV particles of microscopic size which were deposited in a fine layer—like cigarette smoke—on walls, operating tables and other surfaces. When human skin was exposed to the mist, it was susceptible to HIV infection.

Anyone not wearing a mask who entered the room between

surgeries could inhale as much as five micrograms of these aerosolized blood particles—and run a higher than normal risk of contracting AIDS. Unless all surfaces are perfectly swabbed down, even an empty operating room is a dangerous place. What if, in the normal high-speed rush, proper cleansing procedures are not carried out between patients? The study suggests that an infected glove carelessly left on a surface for a few minutes before disposal could deposit the HIV virus on that surface and place at risk anyone who touched it bare handed in the next few days.

But emergency rooms are the most dangerous of all. Says one intelligent agent: "At hospitals like John Hopkins University Hospital, almost fourteen percent of those who come to the emergency room with penetrating wounds test positive for AIDS. The bloodiest wounded pose the most serious threat." A recent study showed that forty percent of all males admitted to emergency rooms in the Miami area were HIV positive.

Even a visit to the doctor's or dentist's office carries a hazard. The Centers for Disease Control does not like to report how many licensed medical personnel are AIDS carriers. But according to the *Medical World News*, as of 1992 there were more than 5,000 dentists, doctors and health care workers infected with the virus. One intelligence agent who monitors the situation places the number at closer to 8,000.

In a study published in the British medical journal *The Lancet* by a team of microbiologists from the University of Georgia led by Dr. David Lewis, the possible transmission of the HIV virus through dental equipment was opened up for scrutiny. The scientists used DNA techniques to identify evidence of the human immunodeficiency virus in two types of commonly used dental tools: the drill and the prophylaxis angle, which dentists use to clean and polish teeth.

The research team tested twelve high-speed drills and forty prophylaxis, and in all cases, they found material containing the HIV virus trapped in the equipment. Dr. Lewis and his team found that HIV escapes the typical chemical disinfectant. "It is usually applied on the outside, which is not enough" said the Lancet report. The substances "were blown out" when the tools were reused, even though they were disinfected with chemical germicides, which suggested a risk of depositing the HIV material in the next patient's mouth. (Similar tests with Hepatitis B were conducted with the same results.) "It truly poses a risk just like a contaminated needle does to a healthcare worker," said Dr. Lewis.

The case of Kimberly Bergalis, a beautiful, 23-year-old who contracted AIDS after a visit to an infected dentist was well publicized by the national news media. Her father, George Bergalis, called Dr. Acer (who died on September 3, 1990) a murderer. "Someone who has AIDS and continues to practice is nothing better than a murderer, that is all they are," he told reporters. "They might as well take a gun and shoot somebody in the head with it."

Kimberly called medical doctors and Acer's colleagues "wimps and bastards," because even when Acer was in the last and most virulent stages of the HIV infection, they allowed him to work, never reporting his condition to the health authorities. Acer was indeed a bastard. He only discussed his condition with the Centers for Disease Control on one occasion, and then, only for an hour. He also destroyed his records. Those who knew him believe he may have been suffering from AIDS-related dementia and intentionally infected Kimberley Bergalis—and perhaps others.

CHAPTER TEN

Despite all the evidence to the contrary, the Centers for Disease Control continue to deny that AIDS infection is possible through casual contact. They preach the gospel that using condoms for "safe sex" will protect the vast majority. But they are playing politics; not practicing science. They deny that the AIDS virus can be found in feces, saliva, sputum, nasal secretions, sweat, tears and urine.*

Yet here is a 1988 report in the Journal of the American Medical Association: "At this point, live AIDS viruses have been isolated from blood, serum, semen, saliva, urine, and now tears," wrote Dr. Restak, a Washington neurologist and AIDS researcher. "As the virus exists in these fluids, the better part of wisdom dictates that we assume the possibility that it can also be transmitted by these routes."

Dr. Restak was right about the better part of wisdom. No matter what line the CDC puts out, the truth is this: the HIV

---

*If AIDS is not found in urine, how does the CDC explain this: On August 1, 1992, a new AIDS-urine test was proven effective at isolating the virus. The test is relatively simple and costs one-third what a blood test costs.

virus can be transmitted by "casual contact." Here's the worst news of all, and it goes directly counter to what the government wants you to believe: Even skin—unbroken skin, no abrasions, no blood—is capable of absorbing the virus.*

Scientists now know this as a result of their work with what they call Langerhan cells. These cells are densely packed in mucous membranes and less tightly concentrated throughout the body. Their function as receptors for irritants on the skin was discovered in Chemical and Bacteriological Warfare labs in 1914 —which led to the production of a substance that was poisonous after settling on the skin: mustard gas.

But the role played by Langerhan cells in actually transporting irritants through the skin was unknown until 1963. What the CAB labs proved is that Langerhan cells attach themselves to the allergen particle, transporting it through the skin to the cell that begins the allergic reaction.

What the Fort Detrick researchers discovered is that Langerhan cells have receptors almost identical to the CD4 receptor cells in the HIV virus. Langerhan cells were mixed with

---

* The campaign to downplay fears of AIDS contagion has been so successful that anyone even suggesting that toilet seats could be dangerous would be dismissed as a nut case. So why, then, did the Fort Detrick virologists conduct experiments with skin cultures to see how many AIDS virions were picked up by the culture after coming in contact with AIDS virus placed on a plastic and a wooden toilet seat?

Those experiments were secret; the intention was that the public would never know about them. But if the government's top scientists wanted the answer to the question about AIDS contagion and toilet seats, then certainly the public should want that answer.

According to the government's own intelligence report about these experiments, AIDS viruses which had already been exposed on toilet seats for four days were potentionally infectious. "Enough virions were found in the cultures," the report said, "to infect a person with a buttock pimple or rash who sat on a toilet seat on which HIV was deposited. All cultures tested showed positive."

HIV virus in a test tube and left for a while. Sure enough, the HIV cells were "recognized" by the Langerhan cells and were able to attach to them.

Then the virologists took live male semen infected with HIV and placed it on clean human skin with no cuts or abrasions. The semen was stained with a fluorescent dye so that its passage through the various layers of skin could be tracked. The Langerhan cells attached themselves to the HIV viruses and transported them in from the surface of the skin. The HIV virus was no longer on the skin, but deep inside the lower skin layers. The fact that Langerhan cells are receptors for allergenic irritants—and more specifically for the HIV virus CD4 receptors—means that it is not necessary for human blood to be present for the HIV virus to be transmitted from one person to another.*

The Fort Detrick researchers, using secret military data from WWI and WWII Chemical and Bacteriological Warfare labs—especially the British labs at Porton Downs, the most advanced facility outside of the Soviet Academy of Sciences at Novisibirsk —also found that "denditric" cells in the mucous membranes of the mouth and nose did not die when exposed to irritants or bacteria.

Instead, they continued passing on the virus. "Denditric" cells, it was found, have the capacity to carry up to 40-45 times as much virus as the targeted T4 immune cells. They become

---

* The proof that these experiments took place—with these horrifying results—will not, of course, be forthcoming. Those who expect "verification" or "source material" to emerge from Fort Detrick are asking the virologists who worked on these experiments to commit career suicide—and maybe worse. Some slight confirmation of the results, however, came from a surprising source in 1991 when Dr. William Haseltine—a strong backer of AZT—admitted what he called "new evidence" that HIV can be transmitted through intact mucous membranes.

virtual continuous transmission belts for the HIV virus. "Dendritic" cells, like Langerhan cells, are found in the sex organs and the anus canal of humans. This speaks for itself about the risk of homosexual activities. No break or tear in the membrane is necessary—nor must blood be present—for transmission of the HIV virus.

If AIDS can be passed by "casual contact," then people must know through testing when they've become infected. At that moment, they become dangerous to others. But the CDC refuses to acknowledge the basic truths of the disease, even denying that—unlike almost any other infection—the HIV virus is capable of penetrating the blood-brain barrier. But intelligence reports on the Fort Detrick research indicate that the virus is able to* hide in "immunologically privileged sites, where T-cells do not penetrate, typically in the brain and bone marrow."

The implications of that simple statement are profound. It means that it is possible that the virus will not always show up in blood tests. People carrying the virus could test negative. Yet the same test done three months later could show positive. A premarital blood test for AIDS would protect neither the husband nor the wife unless it was done at least three months prior to the wedding.

---

* It is an established fact that the virus can ride the macrophages through the blood-brain barrier. Once inside the brain, the infected cells emit enzymes toxic to neurons and immediately begin a toxic reaction.

In *Virology*, second edition, it is proved that the AIDS virus directly infects the neuron and glial cells in exactly the same manner as it infects monocytes and T-4 cells. The same work proves that the GP-120 protein of the AIDS virus envelope inhibits the growth of nerve cells.

Current blood tests are quite reliable at showing infection that is more than three months old. But they are not one-hundred percent reliable. With the possibility of the virus hidden in the brain, there is a small chance of a false negative. "It might be as long as fourteen years before seroconversions show up in tests," the same intelligence report concluded.

The ability of the HIV virus to hide in the brain long before any symptoms of AIDS are manifested is of great importance. It gives the lie to the claims of the Centers for Disease Control—and the World Health Organization—that there is no evidence of a clinically significant increase in neurological dysfunctions among people infected with HIV-I and HIV-II. Their position is that neurological problems do not arise until after immune deficiencies manifest themselves. This is false.

But with such "respectable" scientific support, this view remains the conventional wisdom. That allows authorities to continue their cover-up of the true gravity of the AIDS epidemic. Why? Because the reality is that there are perhaps a few hundred thousand Americans walking around with HIV-infected brains, but manifesting no symptoms and utterly oblivious to their condition—or to the hazard they pose to friends and loved ones and strangers they encounter.

A study at Walter Reed Hospital threatened the conventional wisdom, noting ample documented evidence that the HIV virus has a neurotropic tendency, attacking the brain at a very early stage of infection, long before immune deficiency symptoms appear. Specifically, the study concluded that neurological problems—a persistent headache, lack of concentration and a general malaise which are usually chalked off to stress—are present prior to symptoms of immunodeficiency in about eighty-six percent of cases of those infected with the newest HIV virus.

This is one of the most significant statements ever made on

AIDS (and by no less a hospital than the one charged with the medical care of the president of the United States). But like all other statements that give the lie to the accepted view of AIDS, it was buried and will probably never receive the attention of the media.*

The Centers for Disease Control is America's first line of defense against any epidemic. But its refusal to admit—and publicize—the truth about AIDS makes the CDC part of the problem. Even intelligence reports are not certain how much of that stems from incompetence or politics or personality—and how much is deliberate policy set by those who created the AIDS epidemic.

The Associated Press reported it this way: "Dissension among AIDS experts at the national Centers for Disease Control has led to the suppression of research, sabotaged experiments and the loss of key workers. . . . A former lab expert, who asked not to be named (for fear of reprisals) described how some experiments were tampered with. 'Cultures turned up missing or contaminated and carbon dioxide to virus incubators was turned off, ruining experiments. The internal squabbling eventually led to the departure of key research workers who helped prove blood transfusions spread the deadly disease.' "

The AP report said that the head of the CDC's AIDS program blocked research into a spermicide that could and did kill the AIDS virus within sixty seconds in strictly controlled lab

* The Walter Reed study noted that it was only with the greatest reluctance—and after delaying until December 1988—that the CDC added HIV encephalopathy (a person who is HIV seropositive with disabling cognitive and or motor dysfunction in the absence of a condition other than HIV) to AIDS case definition.

experiments. No trials were done to see if it worked on people as well as culture plates. "There's a long history of bad politics and unhappy people over there," Dr. Steven McDougal, the head of the CDC immunology laboratory told AP. "I can't begin to unravel it."

Perhaps because it wasn't meant to be unraveled. The CDC executive who killed the spermicide program, intelligence reports indicate, did so under orders from the Olympians—who have also made certain that the CDC does not publish or release the true numbers on AIDS and ARC (Aids-Related Complex) diseases in America. Astonishingly, the CDC never issues AIDS statistics that are less than ten years old. You cannot find out from CDC how many Americans have died from AIDS. Try it and see. Call the CDC and ask them: How many Americans have died from AIDS? And see what they tell you.

Even worse, CDC doesn't even keep statistics on those who've died from Aids-Related Diseases. The *Medical Laboratory Observer* magazine has reported that the ratio of ARC deaths to AIDS deaths is "ten to twenty times higher than is ever reported." The CDC has been forced to admit that the deaths may be ten times as great in number from ARC. But they don't know what the real number is.

You have to ask yourself: Why? Why doesn't our governmental institution officially charged with epidemic control make a serious attempt to know—and report—the most important numbers in the deadliest plague America has faced in our lifetimes? Figures compiled by the Rand Institute, which are more current than CDC statistics, conceded that there were at least 500,000 Americans showing fullblown symptoms of AIDS by the end of 1992.

In compliance with various U.S. government and World

Health Organization memoranda, even those Rand figures were deliberately understated by twenty-five percent to fifty-five percent, according to the latest intelligence estimates. The reality, then, is that somewhere around one million Americans were in the advanced stages of AIDS by the end of 1992.

CHAPTER ELEVEN

In the final analysis, people do not die of AIDS. They die of diseases they contract because AIDS has destroyed the ability of their immune systems to fight them off. The AIDS retrovirus goes straight for the central nervous system, as well as the lungs, and it attacks the brain, causing AIDS virus encephalopathy—also known as dementia.

There are three clearly definable stages of AIDS infection. Stage one is the Asymptomatic Carrier Stage. The person may look well and feel well. No sign of AIDS is detected. Stage two begins with sudden drenching night sweats, persistent diarrhea, chronic fatigue, severe weight loss, candidas and psychogenic disorder. These are called Aids Related Complex (ARC) or the pre-AIDS syndrome. The virus has now settled in the brain, kidneys, lungs, liver—even the eyes—and multiplied until its dread presence can no longer be hidden.

All AIDS-Related Complex (ARC) diseases are described as "opportunistic." The most common of these are:

1. Kaposi Sarcoma.

This is an invasive form of skin cancer involving internal organs. "KP" growths occur independently on different areas of the body, and unlike regular cancer, do not spring from an original single cell.

2. Herpes Simplex. (ST)

This disease causes painful severe ulcers in the area around the mouth and perianial areas, often accompanied by bleeding, colitis, cramps and weight loss. When AIDS-related, the disease is often fatal.

3. Cryptococcosis.

When associated with AIDS, this fungial infection causes meningitis, which explains why there are so many thousands of meningitis cases in the U.S. today. Symptoms include stupor, severe headaches, personality changes, facial weakness and double vision.

4. Candidas.

Candidas is another fungi that produces thrush in the mouth, taking the form of thick curd-like white formations lining mouth and tongue. It is always accompanied by swollen lymph nodes and is the precursor of AIDS.

5. Herpes Zoster.

This causes severe skin eruptions, known as "shingles." When AIDS-related, black oozing scabs cover infected areas in the mouth, nose and the anus.

6. Pneumocystis Carini Pneumonia.

One of the ARC diseases most commonly present in AIDS-infected persons. This is a parasitic infection in the lungs, resulting in sharp chest pains, shortage of breath, wheezing and a hacking cough which brings up white sputum. As the disease progresses, the victim feels suffocated. The medical profession, WHO and the Centers for Disease Control have worked diligently to persuade the public that pneumocystis carini is a fairly new phenomenon, but what are the facts?

The National Cancer Institute, well represented at Fort Detrick, knew about this disorder back in 1960, and it is therefore reasonable to presume that it was researched during the AIDS-contaminated smallpox vaccine experiments. Some proof of this is found in the fact that the National Cancer Institute held an important seminar on pneumoncystis carini in October 1976, when it was still a rare disease.

The plot thickens when we learn from intelligence sources that researchers at Fort Detrick discovered that pneumocystis carini could actually activate, or put another way, trigger other viruses. At the National Cancer Institute seminar in 1976, it was revealed that this disease almost always occurred when the patient was already in an immunodepressed state. By apparently back-tracking on all people who had ordered the drug pentamidine isenthionate from the Parasitic Disease Drug Service, a division of the CDC, the CDC said the disease was mainly confined to infants under the age of one and elderly people.

Chronic lymphoid intestinal pneumonia, which is largely confined to young infants under the age of one, was heavily researched and a great number of lab tests were carried out that involved maedi-visna sheep virus. The pneumonia of maedi-visna sheep is very similar to that found in young infants.

Following these experiments, it has become almost routine to find chronic lymphoid intestinal pneumonia in infants who have AIDS. The diabolical connection is not hard to make. In sheep, as in children, the disease is spread by aerosols. Maedi-visna is not a sexual disease in sheep, so obviously, a retrovirus created at Fort Detrick would have to be non-sexually transmitted in order to attack the very young.

* * *

Why is it, then, that this disease suddenly began to manifest itself primarily in the gay community in America?

The suspicion arose that at Fort Detrick a way to contaminate the drug pentamadine isenthionate might have been devised. If so, they would have limited the drug's distribution to one agency. That is exactly what happened. In November 1976, the U.S. Centers for Disease Control became the sole supplier of pentamadine. The fact that pneumocystis is now closely associated with suppressed immune systems should be taken into account here.

CDC suddenly become very interested in pneumocystis carini, and in 1982 reported on blood tests done on three hemophiliacs who had the disease. The CDC report talked about an "education in absolute numbers of circulating T-Cell groups, lack of lymphocyte responsiveness to mitogens, absolute decrease in T-helper cells, relative increase in T-suppressor cells and resultant inverted T-helper T-suppressor ratios."

But what does all that mean? It means that pneumocystis carini closely resembles AIDS. The question then becomes: was this condition somehow artificially induced among the gay population? If so, how was it done? Only those who participated in the Fort Detrick experiments will be able to provide the full answer—and they are not talking. But the latest intelligence reports on the subject indicate that pneumocystis carini viruses were inserted into Hepatitis A shots.

7. *Crytptosporidiosis.*

This is an internal disorder caused by a protozaon such as carried by cockroaches.* AIDS sufferers show a cholera-type

* Most of us have always followed a general rule about cockroaches: if they're spotted in a restaurant, get out. Cockroaches carry thirty different species of bacteria which are harmful to humans. But these nasty insects are now more dangerous than ever. According to intelligence sources who

manifestation of this disease with as much nine to eleven liters of diarrhea per day, severe dehydration and malnutrition.

8. Cytomeglovirus. (CMV)

This is a viral infection which causes terrible lung problems and can cause blindness when AIDS is present.

In Stage three, the terminal stage, the brain becomes dysfunctional, causing loss of muscular control, chronic memory loss, dementia, seizures and the inability to speak in a coherent manner. These symptoms appear in rapid succession, and they are accompanied by often severe psychiatric disorders.

What makes AIDS such a lethal epidemic is that stage one, the asymptomatic stage, can last for years—five years and more is not uncommon. Such persons appear to be in good health, and even remain in good health for varying periods. With nobody sensing danger, they may infect any of their friends or family—or even strangers—because their body begins "shedding" the AIDS virus through bodily secretions, including sweat and tears.

Every person who has contact with an asymptomatic AIDS-infected person is vulnerable. The virus they manufactured at

---

are familiar with the latest research in the CAB labs, cockroaches can also carry the AIDS virus.

In a recent experiment in a secret location (which I can't reveal), as part of a Chemical and Bacteriological Warfare experiment, cockroaches were bred and infected with the AIDS virus. Under controlled laboratory conditions, the cockroaches were starved and then released among penned animals. The cockroaches voraciously bit the animals. All the animals later tested HIV positive.

Cockroaches do bite sleeping humans, so imagine what would happen if millions of AIDS-infected roaches were ever released into slum areas of the Third World and the ghettoes of the United States.

Fort Detrick is much more diabolical than we've been told. Contrary to the numbing lies of the government and the medical profession, you can get AIDS by kissing, from restaurant food, from eating utensils, from bare skin contact—even from performing political acts like cuddling AIDS-infected babies in hospital wards, as Mrs. Bush did during the 1992 presidential campaign. The most notable example was Princess Diana. Remember her visit to an AIDS wing of a London hospital, where she picked up infected babies, shook hands with AIDS patients and then emerged safe and sound. But did she? Will she be safe and sound ten years from now? The fact is: Nobody knows.

It is fashionable to be seen with "Magic" Johnson. Handshakes all around, as well as embraces. When the Australian Olympic basketball team said they would not play the U.S. team if Johnson was a member, the world press tore the Australian coach to pieces. Like Galileo, the coach had to retreat. But Tony Faucci of the National Institute for Allergy and Infectious Diseases has admitted publicly, "we have critical gaps in our knowledge about how AIDS infects humans."

One of those critical gaps is in the food service industry. Americans have long felt safe dining in restaurants, but that era may be passing. But the CDC has done nothing to alert people to the new danger. A large number of persons working in the food service industry are HIV-positive and all attempts to screen food workers for the virus have met with outraged opposition from a number of highly vocal groups who complain about "civil rights" violations. Kentucky is the only state that does not recognize AIDS as a certifiable "handicap" under the Civil Rights Act.

In one state, Michigan, smallpox, gonorrhea and at least five other contagious diseases and any of the communicable diseases on the state health authority list must be reported the moment they become known. Incredibly, AIDS is not on the Michigan list—even though it is contagious and one-hundred percent lethal.

In most states, the law prevents an employer from dismissing a person with AIDS, even if the symptoms are fullblown. This applies to restaurant workers and all workers in the food handling industry. Similarly employees with AIDS cannot be dismissed on the basis of excessive absenteeism nor for excessive health care costs to the employer.

A recent federal statute requires that AIDS "educational" programs be a policy of food processing companies, with the information to be repeated "at reasonable intervals" so that newcomers are aware of the program. But that federal statute also forbids reassigning workers with AIDS to other jobs that would take them away from handling food or waiting on tables.

The question becomes: Why is AIDS being treated as a protected disease?"

CHAPTER TWELVE

The bottom line is this: AIDS is a political disease. Its impact on America is, therefore, being downplayed. Why? Because the perpetrators and the infected share, ironically, a common goal: the less public alarm, the better. The Olympians want the disease spread without interference from a frightened public. People with AIDS understandably want the protection of their civil rights. That could be threatened by a frightened public.

Those who do not want the American public to know the full menace of AIDS deliberately turned the homosexual network into a powerful lobbying force. The gay community has become the unwitting ally of their Olympian enemies. While the Olympians falsely blame gays as the cause of the epidemic, they are still the only ones powerful enough to protect gay civil rights. Their relationship resembles the Stockholm Syndrome, in which the hostages come to feel a strange kinship with their terrorist captors.

The result is a massive propaganda apparatus—with unlimited financing and an efficiently organized gay network—ranged against the American people. The gay network is strong in most countries. As far back as 1978, the International Gay Association

(IGA) was set up—in both senses—in England, with secretariat offices in Dublin and a Gay Financial Center in Amsterdam, which receives large contributions from religious groups, Hollywood stars, and others of liberal bent.

But it is not the welfare of gay men that the IGA has in mind; it is their utter destruction. The IGA has succeeded in getting a number of countries, notably England, France and the United States, to pass laws under the heading of "hate laws" which forbid, on pain of severe penalties, any interference with the "rights" of homosexuals not only to "exist," but to carry on their "lifestyle."

The International Gay Association was responsible for disrupting the International Conference on AIDS in Montreal, Canada. Act-Up members shouted and held up proceedings, while a leader took over the microphone, and in response to chants of "read the demands, read the Manifesto," began to spell out its self-styled International Code of Rights. Here is what the IGA demanded:

1. Anonymous Testing.
2. Confidential HIV Testing.

This was first legislated in California, where the law is now used to threaten doctors with fines of $10,000 and prison if, under any circumstances, they release information on a patient's HIV antibody status.

3. Pre-test Counseling Program.

This is designed to discourage doctors from taking the trouble to test patients.

4. No Mandatory Testing.

In preventing mandatory testing, the gay lobby is actually helping the spread of the disease.

5. No Quarantine Under Any Circumstances.

This harms everybody, including gays, because it allows persons with AIDS to knowingly continue spreading the disease. Stories abound of people who have done just that. The most famous case was the Canadian airline male flight attendant—'Patient Zero," as he came to be called—who promiscuously infected homosexuals in Europe, the U.S. and Latin America, and who, when asked to stop, simply refused. He continued this practice until his appearance prohibited it. There were no legal sanctions to stop him from his monstrous form of mass murder.

6. A Policy of: No Casual Spread of Infection.

The Gay Lobby demanded that government agencies officially adopt such a statement to allay the fears of the public. In other words, it would become the duty of the government and the medical profession to keep the public persuaded that it is impossible to get AIDS from kissing—or any other contact less intimate than sex without condoms.

7. No discrimination (including in jobs or housing).

International education programs in comprehensive sex information supportive of all sexual orientations, describing "safe sex" and needle use practices and other means of preventing HIV transmissions.

The Gay Media Task Force is a committee that reviews television programs about AIDS. This group can make life uncomfortable for any network that doesn't toe the line, as NBC found out in December, 1988, when they screened "Midnight Caller." Rioting broke out in San Francisco, and NBC promised never to ignore the committee again.

The Gay Task Force virtually controlled the dissemination of information about California's Proposition 102, which would have required physicians in the state to report to health authorities all positive HIV tests. It also called for mandatory tracing of sexual partners or intravenous drug-using partners of those who tested positive. The Proposition was voted down with the help of Congressman Henry Waxman and Willie Brown, speaker of the House in the California State Assembly, and the Hollywood crowd.

President Reagan fared no better than NBC. In 1987 the President circulated an urgent recommendation to every Republican governor that they do all that they could to stop the AIDS epidemic. Reagan wanted mandatory AIDS testing. The gay lobby leadership swung into action, and the Surgeon General of the United States, Dr. Everett Koop, personally went to those states with Republican governors and lobbied hard among local and state authorities, urging that the President's appeal be ignored. He persuaded them that mandatory AIDS testing was not necessary to control the epidemic.

When an honest history of the AIDS plague is written, it will be recorded that a small number of people and groups—with billions of dollars at their disposal—were able to persuade the public that mandatory AIDS testing was of no value—and perhaps harmful. Among those listed will be Dr. Koop, the Gay Lobby, the ACLU, the media, the National Organization of Women and Dr. David Axelrod.

Dr. Axelrod is typical of the gay lobby's allies in hindering any progress toward stopping the AIDS epidemic through mandatory testing. With no special qualifications, he was given the position of New York State Health Commissioner—which he owed to his supporters in the Council on Foreign Relations, an Olympian group.

One of his first actions in his new job was to forbid doctors from performing routine HIV tests in their offices. Axelrod gave no reason for his dictatorial edict, which stated that "henceforth all HIV testing shall be done only in special laboratories, those with blood and tissue banks, state, county and or city laboratories located in hospitals affiliated with medical schools, the American Red Cross or New York blood programs, or research laboratories doing public health work under contract."

There was no sound reason to prevent doctors from testing for the AIDS virus in their offices, but Axelrod forced them to send their patients elsewhere at the cost of time, trouble and expense. Why? Intelligence reports say that the gay lobby, itself influenced by the Council on Foreign Relations, was determined to slow down or stop HIV-testing.

Dr. Axelrod's other contribution to the epidemic was his anonymous testing program. At least three-hundred thousand samples were to be collected from hospitals all across New York State, but no names were to be associated with the samples. If a sample was positive, the infected individual could go right on infecting others.

How did Axelrod justify his policy? "We need more accurate information about the numbers and distributions of individuals already infected with the virus," he said, "to plan the necessary medical services and to do extensive anonymous testing, to gather the statistics, but not to stop the epidemic." That was a preposterous statement from a doctor sworn to save lives. Of what value was anonymous testing? None.

But Axelrod was not alone. The medical profession was equally committed to preventing mandatory testing. The *New England Journal of Medicine* and *The Journal of the American Medical Association* both ran a concerted drive against it. Both of these prestigious medical journals made the false claims that widespread testing would give too many false-positive results, causing public panic. The American Medical Association, without the slightest proof to its claims, argued that the false-positive results would "alarm" the public.

Dr. Axelrod and the gay lobby—and the medical journals—simply swept under the carpet the impressive work of the U.S. Army in eliminating false-positive HIV tests. In June, 1986, the results of the Army's mandatory testing were released to the Second World Congress on AIDS. The false-positive results were so low as to be statistically irrelevant.

Colonel Donald F. Burke was the officer in charge of administering the HIV-tests to recruits. His meticulous record keeping has never been questioned, nor the credibility of his report that there was only one false positive test per 130,000 recruits. Even more striking was Colonel Burke's report that by 1983, the Army had developed techniques which cut the rate of false-positive tests to one in a million.

Why have the gay lobby and the Olympians gone to such lengths to prevent mandatory testing? Because they want the public kept in ignorance about how widespread AIDS has become. Mandatory testing would reveal to the public that AIDS is much more widespread than now believed. The Olympians do not want AIDS slowed down by informed public demands for proper epidemic controls.

There is no merit to the argument that a law requiring mandatory AIDS testing would lead to the violation of gay civil rights—or that gays would become the target of an incensed population. The U.S. Army has shown that testing for HIV can be made simple, non-intrusive and highly accurate. The idea that a fatal disease must not be identified in a carrier because it might lead to a deprivation of his civil rights is simply bizarre.

Yet the gay lobby persists in its destructive course. The International Gay Alliance has grown bold enough to ask for "observer status" at the United Nations. A number of U. N.

delegates, including the American delegation, are acting as "ex-officio" representatives for the International Gay Association, thus making AIDS even more of a political issue—rather than a fundamental life-and-death matter of epidemic control and public health.

The gay leadership wrongly—a fatal mistake—believes it has the sympathy and protection of government. Undoubtedly that is true of many compassionate people who work in government and are as unwitting of the real cause of AIDS as anyone else. But the truth about some of those powerful enough to manipulate government at the highest levels—The Olympians—is exactly the opposite.

To the gays, I say this with my deepest conviction, after years of researching the AIDS epidemic: government is your enemy, not your friend. Relatively useless laws passed to protect gay civil rights are nothing but a red herring to draw attention away from the real problem. The real solutions to the AIDS epidemic —for everyone—do not lie in the current policies. Much of the leadership of the gay community does not appear to have grasped this nasty truth. Gays are being duped by a government that has targeted them for death.

To those who would ask: "Is that even possible?" I would say: Look very closely at what the top virologists and microbiologists in the world were secretly discussing with each other at the Banbury Conference in the spring of 1985.

CHAPTER THIRTEEN

On April 28-May 1, 1985, the Banbury Conference on Genetically-Altered Viruses and Environment was held at Banbury Center Laboratories. Banbury Center is the former Eugenics Records Office in Cold Spring Harbor, Long Island. The old Harriman laboratories, which began in 1904 with eugenics experiments designed to create a "perfect" white race and worked for the destruction of blacks and poor whites during the pellagra scourge and opened its facilities to German Nazi scientists during the Thirties, hosted this event.*

The world's foremost molecular biologists and virologists assembled for a conference on: the epidemiology of viruses altered by man. While ostensibly held under the auspices of the Cold Spring Harbor facility, the gathering was carefully supervised and monitored by the U.S. government. At the instruction of several U.S. intelligence agencies, the proceedings deemed sensitive were held under conditions of strict secrecy.

---

* Cold Spring Harbor is the site of frequent gatherings of the scientific elite. See APPENDIX B for a summary of their 1983 conclave. See APPENDIX C for a look at one of their internal documents and an intelligence report about their work.

The official sponsors of the conference were almost all multinational corporations—or their private foundations—with close links to the Olympians. The roster was as follows:

IBM.
The Grace Foundation Inc.
Texaco Philanthropic Foundation Inc.
The Chevron Fund.
The Dow Chemical Company.
Exxon Corporation.
Phillips Petroleum Foundation Inc.
The Bristol Myers Fund Inc.
Rockwell International Corporation Trust.
The Procter and Gamble Company.

These organizations all donated large sums of money for future research. The U.S. government also contributed a substantial amount of money, although the exact amount could not be determined. Letters of inquiry about this use of taxpayer funds, addressed to the General Accounting Office, went unanswered.

Other corporate sponsors who donated various sums of money were mainly drawn from the Olympian network, and for this reason, they are significant:

E. L. du Pont de Nemours and Company.
Hoffman-La Roche.
Monsanto Company.
Agrigenics Corporation.
Beckton Dickinson and Company.
Ciba-Geigy Corporation.
Genetics Institute.
Johnson and Johnson.

Schering Plough Corporation.
UpJohn Company.
Genentech Inc.
American International.
Biogen S.A.
Eli Lilly and Co.
Pall Corporation.
American Cyanamid Company.
Cetus Corporation.
Pfizer Inc.
CPC International Inc.
Mitsui Toatsu Chemicals Inc.
Smith Kline and French Laboratories.

Nearly all of the above are top companies in the pharmaceutical industry or leaders in genetic research. All are connected in one way or another with David Rockefeller, the Harrimans and the Morgan Banks.

In the spring of 1985, the American public was not yet concerned about AIDS. The President of the United States had never spoken the word publicly. It was still regarded as a curse upon drug addicts and homosexuals. Most Americans believed that their odds of infection were about the same as hitting the lottery. Rock Hudson was still alive. It was his death that October that shocked the national media—and the public—into asking serious questions about this thing called AIDS. The notion that it was created by human hand was nothing more than sick fantasy.

Fact or fantasy? You decide after reading E. D. Kilbourne's paper "Epidemiology of Viruses Altered By Man" presented to the Conference. Kilbourne went into great detail about what he called a "maximally malignant monster virus," (MMMV) which he stated could be created in spite of the difficulties that would be encountered in synthesizing it.

His paper was, in effect, a mere confirmation, although he posed it hypothetically:

"Because we know the primary structure of many viral genes and have the technical capacity to synthesize both genes and gene products, it would appear that planned design of friendly or unfriendly viruses is not too remote a possibility. If the latter should be the perverse goal of our paranoid society, can we construct a virus worse than rabies virus with its 100 percent fatality rate or influenza with its pandemic potential for twenty million deaths worldwide? Hypothetically: yes.

"But if the creation of MMMV is unlikely to the point of absurdity, we must also appreciate that in the proper setting single base changes may be sufficient to significantly influence viral properties, including virulence.

Then in an amazing revelation, Kilbourne seemed to come close to admitting that AIDS was indeed a created retrovirus, although he did not actually name it: "The more imaginative vistas of genetic engineering are concerned less with the modification of existing viruses than with the segregation and manipulation of single virus genes. Perforce, the epidemiology of virus genes in new environmental or even different temporal context must be considered."

In other words, the creation of new retroviruses was what appealed to the most advanced microbiologists. Kilbourne then issued a warning that the freezers of most laboratories "are potential if unlikely sources of new pathogens . . . Manipulation of the genes of viruses capable of genetic reassortment must not be undertaken without awareness that these viruses comprise an extended genotype or gene reservoir available for interspecific viral gene transmission."

Research of this nature was precisely what was done at Fort Detrick and Los Alamos and Cold Spring Harbor. One of the most telling admissions during the Conference came when it was disclosed that the purpose of genetic tinkering with the envelope of the HIV virus was to broaden the range of target cells for infection.

Dr. Robert Gallo, the head of AIDS research for the National Institutes of Health, attended the Banbury Conference and felt safe enough to admit, in a moment of spontaneity, that deliberate genetic tampering with viruses had created new, unnatural lethal viruses. In the discussions that followed the presentation of a paper, "Genomic Variations of HTLV-III/LAV, the Retrovirus of AIDS," co-authored by Beatrice H. Hahn, George Shaw, Flossie Wong Staal and Gallo himself, one of the delegates, H. Fields, asked the following question:

"If you took the HTLV LTR's or the region involving transcription and put it into other retroviruses or other viruses, would you have any concern about it in terms of the hosts or the environment?"

As if unthinkingly, Gallo blurted out: "It is already being done."

In plain language, what Fields was asking was: "If we made dangerous new viruses, would you be worried about it?"

Fields followed up by asking: "What would be the nature of your concern, considering everything you have done?"

As a scientist regarded (wrongly) as a world-class microbiologist, Gallo was supposed to be doing everything in his power to stop the march of AIDS. He answered: "I am not overly concerned about attaching the HTLV-III LTR to the genome of other retroviruses because there is much evidence that the cytopathic genome of HTLV III does involve the need for specific regions of the HTLV genome. I would be concerned about doing things that broaden the range of target cells for infection or if something we've done to alter the envelope gives it greater capacity for survival. I would be concerned."

If something we've done to alter the envelope gives it greater capacity for survival. I would be concerned.

He went on to say: "Incidentally even HTLV-I is spreading in many parts of the world because it has a very long latency period and only a 1:100 disease-to-virus infection ratio. It is much less evident, but I suspect HTLV-I is going to be an increasing problem 10-30 years from now. In summary, I would evaluate each planned alteration carefully."

I would evaluate each planned alteration carefully. Gallo's own words can lead only to the conclusion that the alteration of the structure of viruses was ongoing in 1985, and already far advanced. At a closed session of the proceedings, discussions were held about the research of a group of British doctors who wrote a paper stating that they had found the answer to why certain people appear to get AIDS more readily than others. It was in the genes.

Doctors Lesley Jane Eales, Keith Nye and Anthony Pinching found the method of isolating the right gene that resists AIDS and the gene that does not. This should have been an important landmark in AIDS research, qualifying the doctors for the Nobel Prize. But instead of world-wide recognition for their astounding achievement, Dr. Pinching, leader of the team, was forced to withdraw the group's findings on the specious grounds that "an error was subsequently discovered and some of the data was flawed."

The three British pioneers had to be forced underground. Their findings would have caused political explosions around the world. Even the layman would have understood why Africa and Brazil and Haiti were being ravaged by AIDS, while the disease was not spreading as rapidly in Western Europe and the United States: the British scientists had discovered that the AIDS virus attacked the GC-1 gene, common to blacks and "coloreds," more redily than the GC-2 gene common to whites. This would explain why blacks and Hispanics in the U.S. are contracting the disease at a much faster rate than whites: They're genetically more susceptible to HIV.*

* In addition to what we know, there is a great deal of informed speculation—too much to ignore—that Cold Spring Harbor labs are currently engaged in molecular research to develop a virus with even greater ability to infect people who have the most melanin in their skins. Black and "colored" skin has substantially more melanin than white skin. British microbiologists at the CAB research unit at Porton Downs are believed to have successfully developed a virus with a ninety percent selective capability. The means of "steering" the HIV viruses, or indeed any virus, to selected groups, is known to be one of the research programs being conducted at Cold Spring Harbor.

This suits the policies of the International Monetary Fund in forcing greatly lowered standards of living in certain poor countries, whose nationals have been classed as "defectives" by the Olympians. Remember this: most of these countries have valuable natural resources. With the IMF destroying the living standards of these "useless eaters," and a virus capable of attacking people based on the melanin in their skins, is it any wonder that Africa is today almost totally ravaged by AIDS?

The evidence is strong enough that AIDS was designed and engineered to specifically infect blacks that in February, 1989, Samuel Evans, Chairman of the National Council of Public Auditors, called upon the U.S. Senate to investigate ethnic-race specific biological warfare weapons. That means weapons aimed at the elimination of specific groups, including blacks and other nonwhite populations in the U.S..

Evans charged that Colonel David Huxoll, who at the time was commander of the U.S. Army Research Institute for Infectious Diseases at Fort Detrick, Maryland, was allocated $60 million for research into biological ethnic weapons. Evans was apparently aware that Fort Detrick is an important AIDS research facility, because he raised the roof among black Congressmen and political activists. He further charged that Zaire was targeted by the U.S. for AIDS epidemics and that twenty to thirty percent of Zaire's population became infected with the AIDS virus as a result of that experiment.

The report of proceedings at Cold Spring Harbor betrayed their true arrogance. Their conclusion was that the world would never believe that the AIDS virus was the result of genetic reprogramming. There was nothing to worry about. The public should just continue to be told that the creation of such a dangerous retrovirus belonged in the realm of the absurd. Any attempt to open up the truth about genetic tampering—which led to the birth of the AIDS virus and others yet to emerge—would simply be denied and explained away. (Which is exactly what has happened ever since.)

A year after the Banbury Conference, in 1986, there was, as one intelligence report described it, "a further gathering of the initiated at Cold spring Harbor." They were there to hear Professor W. Bodmer of the Imperial Cancer Research Institute, a world-renowned Oxford geneticist, speak on "The Molecular Biology of Homo Sapiens."

Here is a quote from the intelligence report: "Behind closed doors several delegates expressed the view that population explosion was the greatest threat to the stability of the world, echoing the words of Sir Julian Huxley* Harbor Conference: "population growth is the most alarming problem and loss of genetic quality must be reversed."

"Professor Bodmer began his address by saying: 'Analyses of normal human variability in facial features, character and mental abilities is surely one of the real challenges of human genetics.

* Britain's foremost eugenicist of the post-WWII era, who in 1947 was the founder of the "population control" program of the United Nations. In 1951 Huxley consulted with John D. Rockefeller III, General Maxwell Taylor, William Draper and others, and by 1952, a "Population Control Council" was established. In 1966 the name was changed to "Population Crisis Committee." Since 1966, U.S. foreign policy has stressed the importance of "population control," as has the National Security Agency, the World Bank and the International Monetary Fund.

Now, with the availability of polymorphic DNA markers, there is a well-defined approach. The DNA technology that is now available should in due course be able to answer the question as to whether indeed the genes that control facial features and certain aspects of behavior are closely linked . . . Knowledge of the total human genome sequence has profound implications, not only for the analysis, prevention, and treatment of disease, but also for the better understanding of normal variations, and through that, hopefully, making a contribution to solving broader problems of society.'

"Behind closed doors, Bodmer left his listeners in no doubt that one of the greatest 'broader problems of society' was overpopulation of the world by 'undesirables,' and population explosions among black nations urgently needed to be arrested and stopped altogether, and their populations drastically reduced. Although the word AIDS was not mentioned, the sum and substance of Bodmer's remarks left his audience in no doubt that genetically-engineered retroviruses were the only hope of achieving the desired goal."

But the top scientists in the most powerful institutions were hard at work on those genetically-engineered retroviruses.

CHAPTER FOURTEEN

"It is already being done."

"If something we've done to alter the envelope gives it greater capacity for survival."

"I would evaluate each planned alteration carefully."

—Dr. Robert Gallo
Cold Spring Harbor, 1985

All along, the establishment's AIDS "hero" has been Dr. Robert Gallo of the National Cancer Institute. Described for years by the press as the "co-discoverer of the AIDS virus" and "the nation's leading AIDS researcher," Gallo has argued ferociously that AIDS cannot be spread by casual contact of any kind. He has led the way in ridiculing "alarmist" beliefs about the transmission of the disease.

But Dr. Gallo's own credibility has suffered severely in the last few years. Dr. Luc Montagnier of the Pasteur Institute in Paris has always contended that his early laboratory test results were stolen by some unknown Americans, and that Dr. Gallo could not, and did not, isolate the AIDS virus in 1982. A committee of inquiry was called by the National Institutes of Health to investigate several aspects of Dr. Gallo's research.

Among the most important questions about Dr. Gallo:

1) When did Dr. Gallo recognize that the researchers working with Dr. Montagnier in Paris had isolated the AIDS virus?

2) How was it possible that the AIDS virus isolated by Dr. Gallo was a genetic twin of the one isolated by Dr. Montagnier in Paris?

3) How can Dr. Gallo explain the impossibility of the two viruses, isolated thousands of miles apart, being the twin of each other, given the fact that AIDS viruses mutate at such a rapid rate? The virus could only have mutated in one place, in Paris or at the National Cancer Institute in the U.S. But not in both places at the same time.

4) Given the fact that the Paris laboratory isolated the virus two years before Dr. Gallo announced his "findings," Dr. Gallo must have kept quiet about his "results" for two years. Why would he have done that?

5) In his original article in Science magazine, Dr. Gallo claimed that the French and American viruses were different viruses. How can he explain that impossibility?

A strong case exists that Dr. Gallo's "records" of his "discovery" of the AIDS virus were a complete fraud. He was in such hot water that it looked like he might face the public disgrace of being forced to return the $303,000 he had received in royalties for his "testing." The controversy over Dr. Gallo's role—or faked role—in the discovery of the AIDS virus had profound implications for the public—which paid little attention. Because if Gallo was dishonest with the press, the public and his colleagues about his claim of "co-discovery" of AIDS, then why should he be trusted in his explanations of how difficult it is to transmit the disease?

Unfortunately, the public will never know the answers to those questions about Dr. Gallo. Once again, the scientific world closed ranks. Gallo's battle with the Pasteur Institute ended in a sordid compromise between himself and Dr. Luc Montagnier. Jonas Salk, the discoverer of the Polio vaccine, stepped in and "brokered" a deal that would allow the scientists to keep their secrets to themselves and protect their professional reputations.

But the whole dirty business was done at the expense of the public. Dr. Abraham Karpas, Assistant Director of Research, Clinical School of Medicine at Cambridge University captured its essence in a letter of protest he wrote to Dr. Robert Windon, Assistant for Health, Department of Human Services, Washington, D.C.: "There is no question in my mind that certain scientists at the National Cancer Institute are responsible for the lost years in AIDS research. You must realize that this resulted in the logarithmic increase in the number of cases of AIDS virus infection both through sexual intercourse and the transfusion of thousands of units of contaminated blood.

"Progress in AIDS research was delayed by a full year while Drs. Gallo and Essex published eight articles on HTLV, the rare human leukemia virus (also known to be the cause of Chronic Fatigue Syndrome), as the cause of AIDS. In the process they prevented directly and indirectly the publication of medical and scientific data that HTLV was not involved in AIDS and that another virus was the cause of this new disease. As a result, many thousands of individuals became infected with contaminated blood and the virus kept on spreading at an accelerated pace.

"Only after Dr. Gallo received the AIDS virus from France and managed to grow it did he change its name from LAV to

HTLV-II and claim himself as the discoverer. In order to justify calling it HTLV-II, Gallo with Wong Staal presented scientific 'data' on the similarity of the HTLV-I and the HTLV-II, which they published in Science and Nature, thereby causing further deadly delay in AIDS research by sending newcomers to this field into blind alleys.

"There is no question in my mind that Dr. Gallo is responsible for the large number of infections especially through blood transfusions during the lost year. . . . I find it amazing that this situation is being tolerated in the U.S.A. Consider that a democratically elected President had to resign because of the Watrgate episode in which not a single life was lost, while Dr. Gallo was allowed to continue to dominate AIDS research with untold millions from U.S.A. taxpayers, many of whom have become infected by the virus due to Gallo's scientific incompetence and ruthlessness."

The news media covered this story perfunctorily. It should have been a major national scandal, but very few reporters bothered to find out what was going on; it was too complex and unglamorous. There was no audience for it. Gallo got what amounted to a free pass from the press. The public remained blissfully ignorant.

Even worse, the U.S. government backed Dr. Gallo all the way. But why? Because of the Machiavellian nature of AIDS politics. Ample evidence exists that Dr. Gallo's approach to AIDS treatment—his so-called "cell blocker" theory—is another one of those "dead ends" into which Gallo is leading researchers. The Walter Reed study, mentioned earlier, states flatly that there are no cells which cannot be infected by the HIV virus. That would make Dr. Gallo's "cell blocker" completely ineffective. But the truth is that the government—ably represented by Dr. Gallo—is not working to save humanity from AIDS; but rather to forward the interests of the giant pharmaceutical empires. And their first interest is selling drugs. It's another matter altogether whether those drugs actually help AIDS patients.

CHAPTER FIFTEEN

How far has the medical world really come toward a prevention or cure for AIDS? The answer is simple: No progress has been made at all. None. Billions of dollars have gone into the pockets of government scientists and bureaucrats and medical researchers and drug companies—and their largest stockholders, including the Rockefellers—and the public today has no greater protection against infection with AIDS than if no research had been done, and a person infected today will still die from the disease with one-hundred percent certainty. The only progress—which has come from those doctors courageous enough to remain in the front lines of this war, despite its futility—is in treatment of many of the most common symptoms, such as pneumonia, that show themselves as the virus works its deadly path through the body. In other words, good doctors who care can now prolong life and diminish suffering. But that's all we have to show after more than a decade of fighting this epidemic.

Intelligence reports on the work done at Fort Detrick indicate that it will not be possible to produce a vaccine against AIDS. A vaccine won't work, because what will work on one strain of HIV will not work on another. The virus can alter itself, simply by altering a single amino acid on its outer shell. The virologists at Fort Detrick have learned that there are almost 10,000 possible mutations of the AIDS virus.

As Dr. John Seale has reported: "The outlook for a successful vaccine is bleak. None is available for lentivirus diseases of animals. Search for a vaccine against infectious anemia of horses for eight years, and against maedi-visna in sheep for forty years has proved futile. Indeed when antibodies to a lentivirus are produced artificially by vaccination, animals die after subsequent infection more rapidly than those which are not. In spite of many successful vaccines, it should be realized that for the majority of viral and bacterial diseases, vaccines do not work.

"No simple, effective, curative drug, like penicillin, will be available for AIDS in the foreseeable future, because once a person is infected, the viral genetic code is permanently inserted into the human genetic code of cells in the brain and other tissues. Any drug which blocks replication of the virus will have to be taken for life. All drugs used so far are highly toxic and expensive. If a cheap, apparently effective drug becomes available, it will take several decades to be certain that it is both safe and effective. Nevertheless, many companies will announce 'promising' new drugs and a 'breakthrough' in the treatment for AIDS for simple commercial motives."

The classic example is AZT.

"AIDS victims are being deprived of the best possible treatment because drugs cost too much," according to an Associated Press story based on an important Congressional report. "The report, issued by the House Government Operations Committee, says it is 'appalling that despite the fact that AIDS must be considered the single most compelling challenge to public health in recent U.S. history, unfortunately neither the president nor the Secretary of Health and Human Services has articulated any national policy." The committee said AIDS victims are being exploited through 'the unnecessarily high cost' of drug treatment.' "

Take AZT. One drug company, Burroughs Wellcome, is making a huge fortune off AZT. The company admitted, in an article in the *New York Times* in the spring of 1994, that their profit was already in excess of $300 million. This is one of the cruelest hoaxes ever perpetrated on a desperately ill group of people who are paying large sums for a treatment that, far from curing or retarding AIDS, is actually helping to kill them.

AIDS patients are taking this costly drug in the tragically mistaken belief that its approval by the Food and Drug Administration (FDA) means that it must serve a beneficial purpose. What AZT's victims are not aware of is that they are using the most toxic drug ever considered, let alone approved, by the government. So horrific is AZT's toxicity that only about half the AIDS patients can tolerate it. The other half must be taken off it—or they die. Harvey Chernov, an FDA drug analyst, recommended that AZT's side effects—including anemia—were too severe to warrant approval. But he was overruled. AZT is one of the worst medical frauds of our time. One former government intelligence agent who used his connections to dig deeply into the secret story of the AIDS epidemic told me: "The AZT fraud is the greatest swindle since old John D. Rockefeller sold raw crude oil as a cure for cancer—and made about as much profit per pint bottle as Burroughs Wellcome makes on one AZT pill."

The fervent manner in which the medical profession and the media defend and promote the use of AZT could lead one to believe that—innocently or intentionally—they are serving a policy designed to murder people. No less than the *Journal of the*

American Medical Association—which receives substantial advertising revenues from Burroughs Wellcome and the pharmaceutical industry—has backed the use of AZT. Thanks to this concerted support, the number of AZT users now stands at more than 25,000 and is climbing steadily, primarily among homosexuals.

Even more obscene is the program pushed by one of the chief promoters of AZT, William Haseltine of Harvard's School for Public Health, who advocates that healthy gays be given the drug as a preventive measure. For whatever reasons, Haseltine seems to have taken leave of his Hippocratic oath (first, do no harm), not to mention his senses. AZT is highly toxic, severely damaging kidneys and liver, killing bone marrow, causing muscle-wasting, dreadful nausea and violent bouts of vomiting as the body tries to rid itself of the poison. It destroys the immune system, leads to leukemia through the destruction of cells and causes cancer. Even the FDA issued a bulletin admitting that AZT is "a potential carcinogen."

The fact is that AZT will hasten the onset of AIDS, not delay it, because of the drug's depressive effect on the human immune system. Burroughs Wellcome cannot supply data on the cumulative, long-term effects of AZT—and no wonder. Where would they find enough long-term survivors to tell the tale? The U.S. Army has conducted tests that concluded that AZT is largely ineffective as a treatment for blacks; it only aggravates symptoms in the majority of black patients.

Dr. Michael S. Gottlieb says that individuals exposed to HIV "may be subjected to the adverse effects of AZT without proof that it is effective in these circumstances." Dr. Peter Duesberg of the University of California at Berkeley puts it more bluntly: "AZT is incompatible with life." Here's the simplest—and most honest—way to put it: AZT is a killer drug. Why, in God's name, would anyone who was healthy ever consider using AZT? Certainly nobody would, unless it was advocated by a medical "authority" who presumably knew what was best for them.

How the FDA could have passed AZT is a mystery, unless, of course, as several researchers have concluded, the fix was in. For AZT is as expensive as it is deadly. The cost for one year's dosage is about $10,000—if the patient lives that long. (That cost, incidentally, is about half borne by the U.S. taxpayer.)

The FDA didn't even try to protect people. AZT received a virtual free pass through the FDA testing process—and was approved faster than any other drug in the history of the FDA. Given the labyrinthine difficulties of winning approval for even the most beneficial drugs, what happened with AZT could be described as nothing short of miraculous. The mystery of why is deepened by the fact that Burroughs Wellcome, which hadn't participated in the drug's development, was awarded sole and exclusive rights to AZT. There's a scandal of monumental proportions waiting for the first enterprising reporter or Congressman with the tenacity to bring forth the whole truth.

Beginning in April, 1986, AZT tests were launched by the FDA in 12 medical facilities across the U.S. Under the code name "Phase 11," the tests were supposed to be "double blind, placebo controlled," but turned out to be an almost worthless mess of uncorrelated data signifying, at best, utter incompetence —at worst, complicity.

Placebo testing was invalidated because of AZT's horrible side effects. The patients knew what they were getting; AZT is so toxic there is no way to conceal the horrible taste. And no one could have failed to know which patients had the placebos—they were the ones who weren't vomiting. Even more glaring, doctors administering the tests soon discovered that there were substantial blood-profile differences between AZT users and those who received placebos; AZT showed up as the cause of a depression of some blood elements. The two doctors, Dr. Reichman and Dr. Fischl, most responsible for the tests did not inform the medical profession or the public that the tests were totally unblinded.

One of the 12 centers was in Boston. An FDA inspector was shocked by what she found in the tests. There were, she reported, "multiple deviations from standard protocol procedures." So bad were these "deviations" that she recommended the Boston test data simply not be used in the study. She was overruled. On the administrative side, the forms provided to record symptoms were so badly designed that data could not be properly analyzed—and had to be discarded. An FDA inspector noted that in several instances, reports were altered without explanation as to why. (Critics charged that this data was falsified after the number of deaths and serious adverse side effects became apparent.)

One group of twenty-three AIDS patients were treated for less than four weeks, rather than the required twenty-four weeks. For the remaining twenty weeks of their uncompleted test period, statistical projections about this group were no more valid than guesses. The discrepancies discovered at the twelve centers were so outrageous that the "Phase 11" tests were summarily halted before completion. And on and on and on.

An emergency FDA meeting was held to discuss these anomalies and, incredibly enough, a decision was made to retain the false data. Why? A secret intelligence report on the FDA's machinations states that they decided that "retaining the (false) data didn't really change the results very much." But how would the FDA know this? The answer is: It wouldn't. In other words, they would treat this as if they were the Queen in *Alice in Won-*

derland. The results would mean whatever the FDA wanted them to mean.

The media, of course, hyped by government officials, defended the FDA with the seemingly humane rationale that it would have been "unethical" to withhold AZT from dying patients while the normal testing procedure for approval was carried out. The media had no way of knowing the real facts: Between eight and twelve percent of the 4,805 AIDS patients treated with AZT died during the first seventeen weeks of the trials. Faulty data-keeping made it impossible to determine whether that was better or worse than a similar group of patients who were not treated with AZT.

Yet, for some reason, none of the patients who died during the test were given autopsies. This would surely amount to criminal negligence if it were a case involving an individual doctor or the county medical examiner. What possible legitimate reason could there have been for consistent failure to conduct standard autopsies? The FDA refuses to answer all inquiries. Not even the the intelligence agents who tried to answer that question were able to discover much. That is a secret the FDA has successfully kept to itself—so far—even stonewalling the question of where and when the patients on AZT died.

After Phase 11 tests, the FDA completely lost contact with 1,120 patients in the program—didn't even know where they lived, or whether they were still alive. To solve this glaring deficiency, the FDA announced they would rely on "statistical projections" about the status of those 1,120 patients. In other words, the FDA would simply guess what happened to them. And that would serve as reality. Generously, the FDA accorded the 1,120 missing patients a survival rate of seventy-three percent—and the *Journal of The American Medical Association* duly reported this "fact," whereupon it became conventional wisdom for most of the medical profession.

Even researchers who have supported AZT have been forced to make damning admissions. In their book, *AIDS: The Deadly Threat Revised and Expanded,* which was partly based on the fraudulent report put out by Burroughs Wellcome, Alvin and Virginia Silverstein stated: "AZT and other drugs that have been found to be effective against the AIDS virus generally work at the stage when the virus is reproducing actively and bursting out of infected cells. The virus lurking in bone marrow, brain, or skin cells, however, may be more resistant to the action of the drug. That is why AZT can slow or halt the progress of the disease, but is not a cure. It leaves a reservoir of dormant virus that can break out later if the drug is stopped."

Not to mention the risk of cancer. An early FDA bulletin, before Burroughs Wellcome exerted its full influence: "AZT induces a positive response in cell transformation assay, and is therefore presumed to be a potential carcinogen." Subsequent studies confirmed that AZT did indeed cause cancer in animals.

In their favorable report, even the Silversteins were obliged to acknowledge this deadly detail. "The side effects of AZT, too, are worrisome," they wrote. "A new dimension was added to these worries by two reports suggesting that AZT might cause cancer. . . . Then in mid 1990, doctors at major AIDS treatment centers reported a steep rise in cases of non-Hodgkin's lymphoma (an aggressive cancer of the lymph nodes) among AIDS patients taking AZT."

The Silversteins put a charitable spin on that bad news: "There is no evidence that AZT is causing lymphoma. Instead, doctors believe that AZT is allowing people with weakened immune systems to live longer, thus increasing their chances of developing opportunistic cancer."

So there you are. AZT offers AIDS patients the chance to pay $8,000 to $10,000 a year for a drug that will make them horribly ill, damage their immune system, cause kidney, liver and neurological damage—not to mention the risk of cancer—while leaving them with a "reservoir" of AIDS virus ready to burst out at any moment to overwhelm a considerably weakened body.

Despite its negative impact, AZT has now been joined by a newcomer, DDI. DDI is even less effective in stemming AIDS than AZT. DDI is another cruel hoax. So far there is absolutely no evidence that DDI is effective against AIDS. What the evidence does show is that DDI is even more toxic than AZT! Sixty-three percent of those on DDI, according to the American College of Gastroenterology, were suffering severe pancreatitis. The side effects of DDI will far outweigh any supposed benefits to AIDS patients.

But the drug scam continues. With science now poised to enter realms of genetic engineering never before imagined, there is astonishing hope for the fortunate, but greater danger than ever for the unwanted. The future will be a very treacherous place, indeed.

CHAPTER SIXTEEN

Brian Brewer of the world's largest biochemical research complex, the National Institutes of Health outside Washington D.C., states: "We live in exciting times. We are beginning to understand disease at the molecular level." Jergen Drews, head of Hoffman La Roche's research departments, says: "In order to understand what kind of a revolution is underway, you must visit the labs of the drug companies or universities." Herwig Brunner, who heads biotechnology at Boehringer Mannheim, another pharma ceutical giant in the mold of Hoffman La Roche, says "What they are doing is gigantic."

Just what is it that "they" are doing? According to Frank Morich of Bayer research in Wuppertal, Germany, "growth factors can now be introduced or removed as desired." When arterial walls thicken, it is due to "growth factors" which are natural substances that order cells to divide and multiply. These are brought to the site of arterial damage by blood cells that release them into the blood stream.

According to intelligence reports, there are at least ten major laboratories in the U.S. alone working on a method to deliver growth factors in the human body, using microviruses introduced with them into the blood stream which will cause even more out-of-control cellular replication than the HIV virus. AIDS, as we know it, is rapidly on its way to becoming obsolete.*

Modern genetic technology has given researchers of the 1990s an easier and less costly way to find deoxyribonucliec acid, DNA, the genetic material found in most cells. DNA is the databank containing the genes, the blueprints for construction and maintenance of the human body. These tiny building blocks of life are known as molecules, and they store energy, destroy toxins and convert food into new materials of construction. If just one is missing from the link, its absence will cause many diseases to arise. Conversely, if too many are present, that will cause sickness. (You don't have to be a genetic scientist to imagine the immense possibilities opened up by the knowledge of how to artificially introduce a "block" or an "overproduction" in the molecular chain of command.)

Once biologists know a gene, they know the composition of the protein it creates. According to intelligence reports, the gene is first transferred into bacteria and the genetically altered microbes are then cultured in very large numbers. (The materials used are astonishingly simple: Four glass containers filled with glucose solution for the bacteria, an agitator to prevent the bacteria from forming into clumps at the bottom, and an incubator to keep the mix at 98.6 degrees Fahrenheit.)

After as little as twenty-four hours, the desired protein, which could otherwise be made naturally only inside the liver, kidney or brain, can be filtered from the solution. This method is being

---

* Knowledge has progressed so swiftly that eight years of research into Platelet-derived growth factor—PDGF—done in the 1970s by Carl Henrik Heldin of the Ludwig Institute for Cancer Research at Uppsala Sweden, is today done "as a routine chore."

used to create the AIDS virus—and other plague viruses—more rapidly, and to refine the virus so that it will spread more quickly. They are still working to shorten the "symptom-time," the time between the arrival of the virus in the body and the onset of fatal symptoms. One experiment of this new fast-acting AIDS has already been conducted in a remote area of Liberia, bordering on Sierra Leone. The results, I'm told by someone who knows, were "disastrous."

Other laboratories, according to intelligence reports, are working on a group of proteins called receptors. Receptors protrude from the walls of cells like tentacles and act like a boat dock or landing strip, attracting chemical substances. For instance, it is believed that the AIDS virus will not begin to reproduce until it has attached itself to corresponding receptors on artery walls. Only then does the message go out for cells to begin the reproduction process for AIDS.

Stanford Research and Cold Spring Harbor and other labs around the country, as well as in Europe—particularly in Germany—are working hard to find a chemical which will occupy the receptor sites and do one of two things: Where a cure is sought, one chemical will "blind" the receptor so that viruses cannot "dock" or "land" on them. Where the spread of disease is sought, a chemical which has the ability to trick the receptor into accelerating the "landing" or "docking" process is introduced at receptor sites.

Test results carried out at Knoll A.G., a pharmaceutical laboratory owned by BASF, show that tumors grow out-of-control when the chemical it has produced is introduced to receptor sites. "Most drugs either suppress or activate receptors or enzymes," says Hans Uwe-Schenck, head of Knoll AG, "and we have known about receptors for a long time, but now that we know what the molecules look like, we have a new era in drug research."

A new era in drug research. Now, say researchers, with a chemical that could blind tumor and AIDS cells, these diseases could be controlled—and probably eliminated. But the other, darker side of this research is the equal ease of creating a chemical that will speed up and enhance the growth of the AIDS virus.

Today is it no longer a case of searching through 20,000 substances to find a key that would fit the lock; genetic molecular engineering has reduced the odds to one in ten. With scientists manufacturing receptors in laboratories, and able to see what they look like, the search for a key that will lock or unlock their growth as desired becomes that much easier. In this manner will a more virulent, swifter-acting AIDS virus be introduced, when it's ready, into the mainstream of any population targeted for annihilation.

In the CAB laboratories of the West and Russia, work is proceeding on DNA regulators. Scientists know that every third gene in our bodies controls the design and function of the brain. If they locate the right gene, they can create all kinds of conditions. One lab in Germany is well along in its search for chemicals to suppress or reverse the function of genes that control blood pressure. Millions of people may someday die from chemically induced blood pressure disorders. One Danish lab has come up with a drug that, when ingested or injected, causes terrible and uncontrollable fear.

Researchers have isolated only about ten percent of the genes and proteins that control brain functions, according to Hans Gunter Gassen of the Technical Academy in Darmstadt, Germany, but it is also known that a dramatic breakthrough is near. Russian scientists are doing similar research, and they are as secretive as ever about their own "mind control" projects.

* * *

The next revolutionary step in genetic tampering—which the public should demand to know more about—is the Genome Project. In 1990, the U.S. government provided $1.8 billion in secret funding for the largest project in the history of the world into this type of research. The goal of the project is to totally unlock the entire human genome, deciphering complete hereditary characteristics dating back hundreds of years. Axel Ulrich of the molecular biology division of the Max Planck Institute for Biochemistry in Munich calls this massive undertaking "just the first step."

The goal is to understand every gene within the human organism—and how it works. Studies have already uncovered thousands of hitherto unknown genes, each with its own DNA molecules. The Genome Project will determine how these DNA regions interact in the human body. For beneficial ends? Or destructive ends? "We will be working on all of them," says Ulrich. "By the year 2000, there will scarcely be a new drug on the market for which genetic technology did not play a decisive role."

The Genome Project, which is scheduled for completion in 2005, is perhaps the most revolutionary human endeavor of all time. Once the more than six-million characters of both sets of DNA instructions are deciphered, the human of the future will be either a victim of induced diseases—or extraordinarily healthy. The Los Alamos facility is deeply into research of this kind, as is Cold Spring Harbor—both of which have a long track record of biotech engineering with deadly viruses.

The implications of this for those with the power to protect themselves—and those who are deemed expendable—are staggering; and very easy to figure out. If you're a target, goodbye; if they're successful in time, our grandchildren will be Sinatra fans. In his work, *Biotechnology and the Human Genome*, Dr. Mark Bitensky wrote: "There are profound differences in our susceptibility to the way we respond to drugs, and profound differences in our susceptibility to disease and physical agents. . . . Having this remarkable tool of the human genomic sequence will put us in a position to customize medical care, to become familiar with and to address the individual features of our patients. We would be able to advise them about their own risks rather than the population at large. We would be able to diagnose and treat their illnesses and prevent them from exposures which are inappropriate, in a much more sophisticated and human way. . . . There is the opportunity to deliver an extraordinary level of medical care, a level which addresses individual differences and one which encompasses the complexity of humans."

But there is a dark side to this glowing portrayal. The people who control this information will be able, if they wish, to more precisely target those who are meant for destruction. Although Dr. Bitensky does not mention it, biological intrusions by new artificially created viruses will be made that much easier with genome study. The "profound differences" could be exploited as a weapon of destruction—even against entire races—that are no longer wanted.

Any disease could be manufactured in laboratories having the genome history of a specific person—or group. A genetic printout would reveal changes that could be made in a person's enzymes—to create better health or fatal illness. It wouldn't be difficult. The average human typically carries dozens of diseases —which remain dormant, but when properly aroused would cause immediate or slow death.

Under the Global 2000 blueprint for mass genocide of certain racial and socially "unacceptable" groups, DNA research will play an increasingly important role. In *The Technotronic Era*, Zbigniew Brzezinski told us a generation ago what we should expect. By the end of the 20th Century, Brzezinski predicted, our rulers would have at their call virtually all information about every individual—including his or her DNA. Brzezinski was right on target. The Olympians' progress is already well advanced. The Genome Project is merely their next giant leap for mankind.

Despite its awesome benefits, Project Genome is the most potentially dangerous method of population control yet devised. The ramifications are vast. Genome engineering will provide God-like knowledge to a few—and place more life-and-death power in their hands than ever before imagined. A whole new nation of people is quite possible, and with it comes the danger that at any given time, whole generations could be wiped out in one fell swoop by triggering implanted latent killer diseases. After the work of the Genome Project is completed, the AIDS virus—or any virus—could, at regular cycles, be easily spread to wipe out Bertrand Russell's "useless eaters."

CHAPTER SEVENTEEN

No matter what you believe about the cause of the AIDS epidemic, its catastrophic impact is upon us. Remember Don Rowe's analysis for the *Wall Street Digest*: "Public health officials estimate that 2.4 billion people (half the world's population) will die from AIDS within the next fifteen to twenty years. Economically, the insurance and medical health systems could be devastated in the 1990s. Nothing short of a spectacular medical breakthrough will keep Western civilization from suffering the worst catastrophe in the history of the world."

Is that even in the realm of possibility? What follows is an extract from a government intelligence document. This is not the kind of reporting that you will find among the department store ads in your morning newspaper. This is the kind of reporting that is meant to be seen only by government officials. But it is a perfect example of what they know—and secretly discuss, away from public view—about the AIDS epidemic. If you read nothing else in this book, please read this carefully. And absorb it. And then ask yourself: If this is true, why have I not heard about it from my political leaders and the national media?

I quote: "Fort Detrick studies of recent date confirm what was already believed, i.e., that the genetic changes in the AIDS virus are far higher than previously anticipated. With each cell infection, the HIV virus replicating cycle in that cell will produce new variants, which then adapt to the tissue type in which they live. At the same time, the variants show a greater degree of malignancy, which accelerates as the virus grows.

"Thus it is fully possible that a large number of variants of HIV are presently being transmitted from infected to non-infected persons, and at a much faster rate than was previously anticipated. This lends credence to non-WHO (World Health Organization) reports coming out of Africa, Brazil and Haiti, that the spread of AIDS has reached 'explosive proportions' as the greater the number of persons infected with AIDS, the more rapid is the replicating cycle of the virus.

"Further data collected at Fort Detrick confirms that concentration of AIDS virions in the blood is far greater now than when the HIV virus was first introduced into Zaire. Titers of a million infectious virions per milliliter are being found in increasingly large numbers of persons in the last stage of AIDS before death occurs.

"The African continent, Brazil and Haiti have become the home of new strains of the AIDS virus of increasingly great pathogenicity. Fort Detrick and Los Alamos are presently engaged in examining these new strains of the AIDS virus that, at this initial stage of investigation, appear to have the propensity to spread rapidly through the respiratory system.

"These new viruses, which appear to have something in common with equine infectious anemia, if they can be spread by aerosols, pose the greatest danger to humankind throughout the world, as it will be impossible to confine the spread of such viruses to Africa, Brazil and Haiti. Therefore the sanguine approach of what happens in Africa is really of little cause for alarm in the U.S. is a foolish one.

"There is no reason at present to believe that the new AIDS virus will not be borne across oceans by trade winds. The Spanish flu epidemic* proved conclusively that the spread of viruses by winds was the means of transmission between totally isolated villages and hamlets which had no connection to each other. There is every reason to believe that when this new strain of AIDS virus reaches the U.S.—and there are those who believe it has already arrived—its march across the North American continent will be unstoppable. Homo sapiens may well vanish from the face of the earth forever."

---

* Lord Bertrand Russell lamented the inefficiency of wars. They cost too much to be an economically viable means of population control. But near the end of World War I, there was a grave international epidemic: "Spanish Flu," it came to be called, although it actually broke out near the end of 1918 among North African troops—the majority of whom were black or non-white—and then spread to West European troops, which included the American contingent. In the next few years, the Spanish Flu killed millions around the world.

Like AIDS, there was no precursor for the Spanish Flu; it "just appeared as if out of nowhere," to quote a contemporary newspaper account. Like AIDS, young adults were the hardest hit. Like AIDS, it was a retrovirus capable of rapid mutation. Public health records indicate that members of the same families who died were found to be infected by different strains of the virus. The historian Alfred Crosby said: "Nothing else, no infection, no war, no famine has ever killed so many in so short a period of time."

The epidemic killed more than the war itself, and in one fourth the time —and it did so without costly bills for munitions and property damage. Perhaps the Spanish Flu was just one of those tragic flukes of nature that ravage mankind occasionally. Or perhaps, as some in the intelligence and scientific communities now believe, it was a weapon designed in the Chemical and Bacteriological Warfare labs of one of the World War I combatants which "escaped" and infected millions.

In either case, the words of Acting U. S. Army Surgeon General Vaughn when the epidemic was at its height should be applied to AIDS today: "If the epidemic continues its mathematical rate of circulation, civilization could easily disappear from the face of the earth."

* * *

The AIDS epidemic hasn't even moved into high gear yet. The Global 2000 Committee has for its target 500 million deaths by the year 2010. And while the general attitude of most Americans toward Africa is one of indifference, AIDS researchers have detected that the pattern of the epidemic in the U.S. and Latin America is increasingly resembling that seen in Africa: the disease is now being spread heterosexually. It is no longer found in preponderance among homosexuals and intravenous drug abusers.

It has spread to the heterosexual population of all age groups in a manner which has not yet been accounted for. We had better take notice quickly. As Dr. Thomas C. Quinn of the National Institute of Allergy and Infectious Diseases has said: "Once it becomes an established heterosexual epidemic, it has a potential for rapidly increasing in sheer numbers, like in Africa." And today, in Africa, millions are dead. According to one intelligence report: "Africa has entered the era of depopulation."

All of which is exactly what the Olympians planned. England's Prince Philip, who masquerades as a good-hearted Environmentalist, offered a glimpse into their sensibilities with one of the most disgusting jokes in history: Speaking before the World Wildlife Fund on August 8, 1988, the aristocratic prince said: "In the event that I am reborn, I would like to return as a deadly virus in order to contribute something to solve overpopulation."

He is certainly not alone among environmentalists. The most radical of the well-known groups is "Earth First." One of their spokesmen, David Foreman, was quoted in June, 1987, in European newspapers saying: "AIDS is not a malediction, but the welcome and natural remedy to reduce the population of the planet."*

Secret information recently made available to me states that Robert McNamara—who has now been designated chief spokesperson for the Global 2000 planners—has been ordered to step up his rhetoric against "overpopulation," to condition the world's middle classes to the idea that huge death tolls are inevitable on a planet that is filled to overflowing with humanity.

Watch this scenario unfold before your eyes: McNamara's forum will increasingly become the United Nations. Assisted by a team of U. N. sociologists and anthropologists—and drawing on data secretly provided by Cold Spring Harbor—a blueprint for further genocide was drawn up. Entitled "A Global Policy to Advance Human Development in the 20th Century," it runs

---

* Here is a partial list of leaders of the "environmentalist" movement who have stated that overpopulation is a major problem that requires drastic solutions:

—Dr. Luc Hoffman. Hoffman LaRoche pharmaceuticals.

—John H. London. Former chairman of Royal Dutch Shell.

—Thor Heyerdahl. Explorer, member of the Club of Rome, managers of the genocidal Global 2000 program.

—Robert O. Anderson. CEO ARCO and founder of the Aspen Institute of Colorado.

—Maurice Strong. Chairman of Petro-Canada and Aspen Institute.

—World Health Organization (WHO).

—World Bank. Coined the phrase "appropriate technology," meaning archaic agricultural methods. Leader of the drive to depopulate Africa.

According to theoreticians at Wilton Park, The Tavistock Institute, Stanford Research Center and the Aspen Institute, when the number of people living in cooperation increases, a larger and larger society ensues, thus consuming more and more "scarce natural resources." This is the darkest fear of the Olympians: natural resources being consumed too rapidly by unworthy people.

This is at the heart of "environmentalism," which in the Machiavellian ways of the Olympians has become a well-conceived and executed cover for their plans to diminish the world's population.

fifty-six pages and outlines what McNamara will be telling us. Its thrust is for "massive global efforts" to curb population growth before the end of the 1990s.

The International Monetary Fund also plays an indirect, but very important role in this global genocide plan. The IMF has been accused of creating conditions that are right for the spread of AIDS and AIDS-related complex diseases—particularly tuberculosis, which has always been known as "the poor man's disease.

The IMF lends money to countries with "conditionalities" that the recipient governments are duty bound to follow. The most severe conditionalities fall on the poverty-stricken Third World Countries. An intelligence report on world economic conditions recently stated: "The IMF gets data from applicant countries on their Relative Unit Cost index (RULC), which is a key economic indicator measuring domestic labor costs against international labor costs, weighted in relation to trade by developed countries with underdeveloped countries. RULC is the key to creditworthiness of a country and shows also its need for devaluation where such a need exists. It is the index used to determine whether a country will be in a position to repay its loans through its capacity to generate exports.

"This index and the index used to determine effective exchange rates have been, over the years, systematically rigged by the IMF. In this manner, the IMF is able to put the pressure on governments to cut cost-of-living standards. The policy of the IMF is to demand less and less money be spent internally on health care, food and housing for local populations. In most instances this is complied with. Brazil is a good example, because the cruzeiro is devalued almost every three months and the standard of living of the population reduced proportionately.

"This has led to malnutrition, overcrowding and poorer and

poorer health care. This is the situation that is rife in Africa, certain parts of Latin America and the Caribbean. It is an ideal climate for diseases to be introduced with a cover of natural causes.

"There have been cases where enraged members of governments with large impoverished populations have attempted to expose IMF rigging of key data, but the IMF has dismissed such officials as being ill-informed, while privately threatening those governments with cancellation of loans if any further complaints surface. This has, up until now, had the desired effect.

"Arising out of severe conditionalities imposed on Third World countries by the IMF, many epidemic-type diseases are now flourishing, not the least of these being tuberculosis, of which a new strain that resists known treatment is becoming more common."

Referring to African countries, the report said: "Since implementing the structural adjustment program (conditionalities) laid down by the IMF in 1986, health care has declined sharply, and with it, the number of deaths has escalated dramatically. Yellow fever, malaria and cholera, previously controlled by an adequate health program, are now raging unchecked throughout these countries.

"Nigeria, one of the wealthier counties under the IMF program, is also feeling the limitations imposed upon it. Nigeria has sixty percent of all doctors and nurses in black African countries, but this healthcare force has been steadily cut down since 1986, until today, Nigeria is ripe for a massive outbreak of the traditional diseases which will make it easy for AIDS to spread like wild fire.

"The condom solution is being used by the IMF for the purposes of birth control, and although extensive advertising campaigns were launched to promote their use, the quality of the condoms is so poor that as much as eighty percent of them break or leak.

"The AIDS virus has entered into an explosive phase in Africa, and the same condition is fast being approached by Asian countries such as India and Thailand. By the year 2000, computerized projections show that there will be close to one-hundred million cases of AIDS in Africa, with India and other parts of Asia projected as having a combined total of ninety million cases.

"Projections carried out at Los Alamos indicate that there will be a total of two-hundred million cases of AIDS in underdeveloped countries by the year 2000. There is some concern beginning to surface among the team that the AIDS pandemic may not be stoppable. With seventy-nine to eighty percent of AIDS cases occurring in Third World countries, AIDS may well already be out of hand. There is an acceleration of the epidemic which is matched by a diminishing of responses.

"Almost seventy percent of all AIDS cases in Africa are among heterosexuals. The same holds true for Asia and Brazil. By the year 2000 the number of people in Asia suffering from AIDS will equal those of Africa. AIDS has become the killer of the poor, thanks to the cuts in standards of health care and lowered nutrition standards to meet IMF demands.

"The latest report from WHO which is not being circulated is that governments of poor countries have given up the struggle to contain AIDS. This applies particularly to India, where the AIDS epidemic is exploding with a virulence unmatched in Western countries.

"From the point of view of senior virologists, there is no cure in sight for AIDS. The view taken by Dr. Jonas Salk that a means must be found of boosting the human immune system rather than trying to develop antibodies that can kill the AIDS virus appears to be gaining ground among those members of the medical profession who are realizing that AIDS is a created virus.

"Underlining the findings of how the IMF is affecting the situation, a new threat, that of a highly virulent form of tuberculosis is now taking hold in poor countries and among the poor in the United States. . . . A report compiled by the CDC which is not being circulated says that the incidence of the new drug-resistant strain of bacilli is now twice as high since the last study was done in 1984. Tuberculosis has increased by twenty percent in the U.S. since 1985. Every TB patient is a target for the AIDS virus, and those with AIDS are highly susceptible to contracting tuberculosis. The ramifications are not difficult to comprehend; a twin plague of the most virulent kind is about to explode with great force in the overcrowded inner cities of America, and has already begun.

"To confirm the ratio of tuberculosis to conditions of poverty, a recent study of the homeless was undertaken by a Los Alamos team. The results bear out the "poor man's disease" label in that homeless people are forty times more likely to contract tuberculosis than those in comfortable circumstances. The conclusion drawn is that the spread of TB is accelerating at a faster rate than ever seen before, and that the outbreak of lethal epidemics are at hand."

AIDS is the key to Global 2000 plans, because of its effectiveness in attacking the lungs. Imagine a searing epidemic of AIDS, followed by an epidemic of tuberculosis and then pneumonic plague, like the one that killed hundreds of thousands in Manchuria and eastern India during the period 1910-1911 and again in Europe in 1919-1921.

When the AIDS virus becomes localized in the lungs, it is spread by respiratory discharges, such as coughing and sneezing, and in favorable climatic conditions becomes a highly contagious infectious disease. One of the favorable conditions for the spread of AIDS is crowded dwelling space, inadequate ventilation and the weather, especially when the weather is cooler, as it is during winter in the Middle East, India and Pakistan, Malaysia and the Philippines. Pneumonic Plague would thrive in those conditions.

It is not difficult to envision the rapid spread of tuberculosis in the wake of AIDS, followed by pneumonic plague throughout Africa, given the conditions so graphically described by Dr. Debret in his 1989 *Paris Match* interview, and spreading from Africa to India, the Philippines, Malaysia and China. The United Nations, backed by military forces of the United States, could effectively quarantine these nations, making it difficult for anyone to escape the "cordon sanitaire" set up by the World Health Organization or some other One-World institution. Millions would be left to die. Somalia was a "test case." After a new mosquito-borne malaria that acts against the immune system was released into the population, U. N. troops were sent in to test the "cordon sanitaire."

As this strategy moves forward, loans from the International Monetary Fund and the World Bank to Third World countries will increasingly require governments to enforce specific plans to diminish their populations. Contraceptives and severe penalties for families exceeding certain numbers are a part of this regimen. McNamara will emphasize four global environmental problems created by overpopulation: the loss of bio-diversity, acid raid, the destruction of the ozone layer and changes in the climate.

"All are functions of rising population levels," he has stated, "and increasing consumption per capita." Although he has always neglected to mention that the huge consumption levels that are dangerous to the environment are among the rich; not the poor. It's not the poor of the world who burn millions of gallons of petroleum flying around on private jets. It's not the poor of the world who are burning a hole in the ozone layer. It's not the poor of the world who are bulldozing the Rain Forests to create new wealth. Try to imagine the vastness of the earth's resources burned and consumed to support the lifestyles of any one large clan of superrich—like the Kennedys or Rockefellers or Sabahs of Kuwait—compared to the necessities that sustain the simple lifestyle needs of the poor villages around the world.

As McNamara and his team were working on their Global 2000 plan, the World Health Organization in Geneva was sending out directives to their branches, demanding "a significant increase in the number of viral vaccines without a reduction in quality or potency." The pressure will be on in the second half of the 1990's to speed up the pace at which they rid the planet of its "useless eaters."

The Catholic Church can—and will—use its vast resources to fight the Global 2000 plan for mass sterilization and contraception. But not even the Catholic Church would dare blame the Olympians for the deaths of tens—or hundreds—of millions from "natural causes." The AIDS epidemic will only be a part of that. The Global 2000 Committee is also counting on an epidemic of tuberculosis, which has already infected more than a billion people. The new TB strain is resistant to all known methods of treatment, and the death rate from the new tuberculosis bacilli is ten times greater than from previously known types of the disease. This new strain may well be part of the process designed to "speed up" the death rate. But as long as the world believes that AIDS and this new strain of TB were created by nature, those deaths can only be lamented as the tragic result of "natural causes."

* * *

How many people will allow themselves to believe the truth? How many will demand an honest answer to the question: Was the AIDS virus really created in our own Chemical and Bacteriological Warfare labs?

Perhaps not enough. As Dr. John Seale said: "Doubtless most people will dismiss the suggestion that the AIDS epidemic in the United States may be the result of an act of deliberate biological warfare as worthy only of a fictional plot by Ian Fleming. But it is certainly no less plausible, scientifically, than the hypothesis currently favored by molecular biologists. It may even be true, though strange, but truth is always stranger than fiction."

Dr. Seale sadly concluded: "The greatest coverup of any disease in history is in progress." The participants in the coverup, says Dr. Seale, include the editors of medical and scientific journals who "have misled their professional colleagues about the nature and severity of the AIDS epidemic . . . By selective acceptance or rejection of original papers and letters, and by selecting authors to write 'safe' editorials and review articles, they have perpetuated dangerous misconceptions."

But he knows what his colleagues know: "Every biological scientist who has dispassionately studied the virus and the epidemic knows that the origins of the virus could lie in the development of modern biology, just as the origins of the nuclear bomb lie with modern physics. . . . Most who see it keep quiet, but increasing numbers are talking privately though they still lack the moral courage to speak out in public. They still hope it is a nightmare which will vanish with tomorrow's dawn."

* * *

But the nightmare won't vanish with the dawn. If we pretend it will just go away, the worst is yet to come. And, as Schopenhauer, the philosopher, said, so on until the worst of all. But what can we do? Draconian solutions run against the American character. How many Americans, with their tolerant attitude toward civil rights, would go along with compulsory AIDS testing? For everyone. With the government then enforcing policies that would ensure that the infected do not pass on the virus to the uninfected.

I leave it to each individual's own imagination how that policy would be carried out—and with what impact on our lives, on our society, on future generations, on civilization as we know it. As Dr. Seale has written: "The actions required by government are comparable to those taken in waging a war." In Africa, stern measures to isolate those with AIDS are beginning, although much too late to save the population. And in India, anyone found to have AIDS is immediately imprisoned—and never released. Period.

And yet: The most horrifying thought of all is that if we don't demand from our institutions an immediate and honest response to this epidemic, that is exactly the kind of future that awaits us. If the Olympians are given free rein to spread AIDS under cover of "natural disaster"—and complete protection of all civil rights of the infected—until the gravity of this crisis becomes apparent to all Americans, then that sort of draconian solution is what the mobs in the streets will be demanding.

A plague panic will catapult us into police state solutions—which, for the Olympians, will be a lovely fringe benefit of the AIDS epidemic, since they'll be controlling the police—beyond any nightmare we've ever imagined in America. Remember what Brzezinski told us more than 20 years ago: It's about control. In all its forms.

If the Olympians succeed at keeping the American public asleep until their very survival as a nation requires a police state, then the Olympians will happily step in to run it. And be perceived as heroes for saving the day. Out of this nightmare comes the unthinkable in the early 21st Century: A dictatorship—worthy of a Hitler—running America. And with technology (and biotechnology) in its arsenal that is beyond Hitler's wildest dreams.

CHAPTER EIGHTEEN

We must take action. But what? I don't have an agenda of policies. I'm not a politician. The current debate swirling in Congress over the future of American health care is enough to persuade me that no one person has all the answers. What I do know is this: The right questions must be asked —and honest answers demanded. Any solution to the AIDS epidemic must begin with the public learning the truth about two questions: What caused it? How does it spread?

We are already in a crisis among scientists, researchers and virologists working on AIDS. Almost every laboratory in America is polarized between those who want full disclosure and those who do not. A growing body of researchers, scientists, doctors and virologists abhore the politicization of the AIDS plague and are demanding that the truth prevail.

But this group is not strong enough to make their voices heard in the media. They are ignored. And when they do make their views known, they are threatened with loss of jobs and other reprisals. That must change. Public pressure must convince politicians that they have no choice but to seek the truth about AIDS.

Even the Olympians respond to public outrage. Witness Watergate and the Iran-Contra scandal. It wouldn't take very many Chemical and Bacteriological Warfare scientists testifying before Congress—under forced grants of immunity; talk or go to prison—before even the Olympians would be running for cover.

When they see the public and the press turning against them, they'll become more cautious, perhaps even put some of their grand ambitions "on hold." That alone would save lives. Prosecution of those who created this monstrous plague could permanently remove them from society before they do more harm. And it would put their spiritual heirs on notice that America will no longer tolerate this kind of criminality.

The revelation of some of America's darkest secrets would have a cleansing effect on the political climate—and allow a new debate about how best to cope with the AIDS crisis. Until now, the suffering of those with AIDS has been stressed while the suffering of those who will someday get AIDS has been ignored. We have been lulled into treating AIDS as a civil rights issue, rather than a public health issue. The rights of those already infected have taken precedent over the rights of the uninfected.

God knows I would not want to see more harm come to anyone with AIDS. They deserve the best medical care available, the most compassionate treatment and all human understanding that this disease is not their fault. But those who are stricken do not have the right to infect others. Epidemic control measures must be invoked in industries—health care workers, food service workers, for instance—critical to the public health.

Would we take our children to see a doctor who was visibly infected—showing large pustules on his face and arms—with smallpox? If not, then why should we take our children to see doctors and dentists who draw blood while infected with AIDS?

If our local public health board would crack down on a restaurant that allowed waiters and dishwashers to work with measles, then why would we not demand the same level of confidence that food servers are not infected with AIDS?

This is not prejudice against people with AIDS. This is a straightforward matter of public health. If it takes government insurance, along the lines of social security, to provide an income for those displaced from their work, that is preferable—and ultimately less costly, almost no matter how expensive.

Blood banks must have a strict screening process for all donors, a process that is one hundred percent fullproof, regardless of the cost. But the Council of Community Blood Centers and The American Association of Blood Banks vigorously oppose any mandatory program for screening donors. And the government has taken no action to put severe clamps on who can donate blood—and who can't.

What is urgently needed is a law requiring a sworn affidavit regarding sexual behavior of all volunteer donors, with severe penalties for those who lie. But it is not only gays who are donating contaminated blood. There are hundreds of thousands of heterosexual Americans who have no idea—and no reason to believe, given the misinformation about how the disease is spread—that they are HIV-positive. When they walk through the doors of a blood bank, they are a menace—and they don't even know it. They are unwittingly allowed to spread the epidemic.

We are told that these people must not be discriminated against. The rights of the potential donor are protected; but not the rights of the innocent recipient. No attempt has been made to introduce fullproof screening methods for all blood donors. The debate has centered on civil liberties—the right of privacy—rather than public health. But nobody has a right to donate blood without careful screening to assure that they are not infected with HIV.

This must be perceived as a matter of epidemic control, rather than civil liberties, or the death toll on innocent people will rise to levels beyond what anybody would now believe. This is not only a life-and-death matter for individuals. This is a life-and-death matter for society.

CHAPTER NINETEEN

Is there hope? For you? For me? For all of us? The answer is yes. It lies in "natural medicine." Herbs. God-given plants that have curative powers. The pharmaceutical giants will go on reaping billions in profits selling drugs. But they won't market one that saves the lives of those afflicted with AIDS.

There will almost certainly never be a vaccine that will wipe out AIDS—as there was for polio. The virus is too complex. It has the ability to mutate into thousands of genetic forms. The search for a vaccine will merely squander precious resources enriching yet more scientists and corporations for no human benefit. Many mainline scientists would agree that the chances for an AIDS vaccine in the foreseeable future are slim—and none.

Yet the corporations persist—and pocket the money.* Genen-

---

* The following companies are engaged in "research" to find a cure for AIDS: Biocene, Genentech, Merck/Meddimune, Merck/Repligen, Progenics, UBI and Viogenics. Companies engaged in manufacturing experimental post-infection "therapeutic" vaccines are Biocene, Genentech, Immune Response and MicroGene Sys, while those engaged in experimental drugs for post-AIDS infection are Abbott, Augouron, Bristol Myers Squibb, Burroughs Wellcome (actually Hoffman La Roche) and

tech, which is partly owned by Hoffman La Roche, is, according to intelligence sources, willing to risk even more lives for their products. They are cooperating with the World Health Organization to commence massive clinical trials of new vaccines with uninfected volunteers. One of the new vaccines to be used in this clinical trial is manufactured from HIV particles stripped of their envelopes. The trials are scheduled to begin in 1994.

The World Health Organization will search for volunteers among gays—and other "high risk"—subjects. Each individual will have to make his or her own decision about participating in such a trial. Based on what I've learned, here's the decision I'd make for myself: "No!"

Arab historians centuries ago concluded that medieval healers found a cure for the Black Plague—and those who were rich enough to acquire it were reasonably safe from the death that surrounded them. Historians of the era recorded that the herbal cure had a very high success rate.

Intelligence reports on microbiological experiments at the Institute of Immunology in Moscow speak of a common weed found in Egypt being used to help AIDS patients. The weed is said to be mixed with 8-methoxpsoralen, plus white cells from the AIDS patient and then exposed to ultraviolet light, after which it is injected into the patient's body.

Another intelligence report mentions in passing that the National Cancer Institute requested plant collectors from all over the world to send samples of plants to the Institute. Apparently this request was activated by reports that British scientists were

---

Upjohn. Remember: Included among these corporations are the ones who brought us AZT, DDI and DDC.

working on a compound taken from chestnut trees, black mulberry trees and from tropical legumes, which was showing great potential in treating AIDS patients.

Other reports mention in passing a protein from pokeweed leaves that is far more effective than AZT in inhibiting virus production. A natural compound containing pokeweed proteins enters cells, killing HIV viruses without damaging the cells themselves. (Pokeweed is a weed, with poisonous berries and roots, found in the U.S.)

The only success to come out of AIDS treatment in Africa so far has come from ancient herbal medicine. Now that modern medical science has been seen by Africans as helpless against the onrush of the epidemic, many are turning to traditional herbalists such as Grace Chihuri in Zimbabwe, who says she has the cure for AIDS—and whose successes have led medical people and journalists from around the world to visit her.

Grace works from her crowded Harare apartment, and stores her herbal medicine in old liquor bottles. In her carefully kept redbook of the people she has snatched back from the jaws of death are more than a hundred and twenty names. One of her patients was Sophie Chikondo, a registered nurse who contracted AIDS while delivering the babies of HIV-positive mothers. Two of her friends, both nurses, who contracted the AIDS virus after she did, have died. But the herbal medicine administered by Grace Chihuri caused her diarrhea to disappear and the swelling in her groin and armpit to subside. That was two years ago, and today Sophie is alive and seemingly well.

In the African country of Ghana, Nanan Kofi Drobo was an herbalist who attracted AIDS sufferers from all over the world, particularly Europe. They came to him because of his amazing record of success in healing AIDS cases, using only herbal compounds. Drobo was a man who knew what the Western pharmaceutical companies did not know—or pretended they didn't know. He knew how to stop AIDS in its tracks with herbal compounds.

His success in treating AIDS patients sent fear coursing through the medical and pharmaceutical establishments. Drobo's work was not sanctioned by the Ghanian government, which was under pressure from the International Monetary Fund (IMF) and powerless to disobey the IMF's orders to destroy Drobo's work. In the end, Drobo grew so renowned that he had to be killed. This heinous crime has been officially classified as "suicide by means of self-inflicted gunshot wound."

The weird part is that all of Drobo's herbal compounds—and his formula and notes—were missing from his home when he was found. What happened to them? So far, the Ghanian authorities are not saying.

None of this should be surprising. Western pharmaceutical companies, after all, make much of their profit by chemically synthesizing the healing powers that are naturally present in plants. Whether it's aspirin or digitalis, the beneficial effects come from plant life.

The same is true for AIDS. The cure exists in plant life. AIDS research is not necessary. All AIDS research now is about money: Billions in profits. And the pharmaceutical giants know it. At least one of them is well aware that an herbal formula that cures AIDS has been found and is being deliberately withheld from the world. It will be made available only to the Olympians and their families and friends, just as the Venetian oligarchists found and kept to themselves the secret Egyptian herb formula that kept them and their families and friends safe during the Black Plague of the Middle Ages.

Those who have this herbal formula have every intention of keeping it a secret, and they have the power to enforce that secrecy. Nor is anyone likely—as things stand now—to duplicate their discovery. Much of the expensive scientific research into deliberately steered away from potentially fruitful approaches. Even the best-financed scientific insitutions have been skillfully led down blind alleys.

There's nothing any of us can do to force these people to reveal their herbal treatment. But I can do this much: I can present the information I've acquired about what they've learned, so that virologists and genetic engineers who want to help mankind can finally go down the right path. The logic of what I'm presenting here can be confirmed by any virologist in the world.

The right path is this: What they've discovered is a deoxyribonucleoside. AZT, DDI, DDC and all of the other "promising" drugs use a neucleoside analog. That is to say, they all use a riboside.

Riboside allows the HIV-RNA messengers to invade the cellular membrane to the nuclei of the cell where they replicate in geometrical progression: 2, 4, 8, 16, 32, 64. In an amazingly short time, the numbers become astronomical. That is what makes these drugs that "slow down" the infection worse than useless. The companies that make them deliberately use the neucleoside analog instead of a deoxyribonucleoside, which has the property that prevents the RNA viral messenger from infecting the nuclei of the cell.

Their secret product:

(1) Increases blood platelet integrity.

(2) Increases transmutation inhibition.

(3) Contains sufficient amounts of interferon.

(4) Increases the stem cells.

(5) Contains a co-enzyme which prevents RNA viral messengers from infecting the cell.

For virologists and genetic engineers, the key is in Appendix B, where the Cold Spring Harbor virologists explain what the virus does. The solution is in a product that can stop the HIV from penetrating the cell. (AZT, for instance, does not stop the penetration.) There are plant substances capable of doing this.

That's as much as I can say and hope to stay alive. I've now done all I can do. The rest is up to the scientists who can see that this is the right direction—and are willing to follow it. And to all those who aren't scientists and are willing to pursue the truth on their own. We have been told, and come to believe, lies that are monstrous. Time is now short. Even the intelligence reports indicate that much. Only the truth will save us. If we are to live with hope for our future—and the futures of our children and grandchildren; indeed, civilization as we know it—we must quickly demand that our government and our leaders provide us with absolutely nothing less than full disclosure.

APPENDICES

APPENDIX A

One of the most important investigations into AIDS was carried out in 1988 by the Social Services Committee of the House of Commons in the British Parliament. They were given considerable help, incidentally, by disaffected intelligence service agents and members of the medical and dental professions. The "Third Report from the Social Services Committee, Problems Associated with AIDS, Minutes of Evidence and Memoranda" is of great interest.

One of its quoted documents is a memorandum from Dr. John Seale, Royal Society of Medicine, who has come as close to the truth publicly as any medical authority in the world. What he says contains great wisdom—and the beginnings of solutions that could ultimately save millions of lives. This is an historically important document. I quote it in its entirety.

Dr. Seale:

No politician can make rational decisions to deal with AIDS without a clear understanding of the nature and severity of the epidemic, the means of transmission of the virus, and the prospects of a cure or preventive vaccine. The key scientific facts underlying the epidemic are quite simple, though AIDS is perceived to be unusually complex and full of scientific uncertainties. These perceptions have been produced by a few scientists and others who have recklessly minimized the seriousness of the epidemic and have fostered confusion and dangerous misconceptions.

The most important and urgent task for politicians, both in Government and in Parliament, is to force scientists to speak clearly, precisely and honestly about the AIDS epidemic. Half-truths, wishful thinking, flawed scientific hypotheses and deceptions have been perpetrated by scientists and allowed to flourish as conventional wisdom, aided and abetted by editors of scientific and medical journals. The deceptions must be exposed with maximum publicity.

The public must be fully informed of the true nature of the threat from the virus which faces us all. Once this is done the mass of the population will accept the measures inevitable to halt the spread of the virus, even though they will inevitably require severe curtailment of the liberty and civil rights of everybody, just as happens in war time. The longer the truth is obscured from the public, and the greater the multitude of innocent people who die most horribly as a result, the more ferocious will be the explosion of hatred and revenge against those guilty of perpetrating the deception.

The virus has the properties of a skilled, devious, hidden and implacable invader with the capacity and willingness to kill every man, woman and child in our country. It may be now spreading amongst us precisely because it has this capacity. It is unwise to think that such a force can be vanquished without taking actions which the people of Britain accepted as entirely appropriate in two World Wars; particularly as dissemination of the virus is being actively encouraged by some who wish to destroy our society."

Dr. Seale provided a brilliant overview of the entire situation the world faces in the AIDS epidemic:

A. THE NATURE OF THE DISEASE

1. AIDS is a contagious, infectious, communicable disease caused by a lentivirus (slow virus), a member of the family of retroviruses.

2. No lentivirus has been known to affect humans before the advent of AIDS.

3. AIDS is a typical slow virus with a prolonged, silent incubation period of great variability, but usually lasting several years, followed by slowly progressive disease always ending in death.

4. An epidemic of a new slow virus disease spreading unchecked is the ultimate virological nightmare, yet in none of the major scientific or medical journals has this been spelled out clearly and the implication discussed.

5. Death is caused by the AIDS virus infecting, and slowly destroying, cells in the brain, lungs, intestine and immune system.

B. MORTALITY FOLLOWING INFECTION.

1. Within five years of infection with the virus, twenty-five percent of people have developed fullblown AIDS and all of them die.

2. The ultimate mortality within twenty-five years of infection is unknown as the virus has been spreading for only ten years. The optimistic view held by a decreasing number of virologists is that only fifty percent of those infected will die. Many virologists accept this pessimistic view, that all people infected with the virus will eventually be killed by it.

3. All virologists are agreed that once infected with the AIDS virus, people are potentially infectious to others for life.

C. FAILURE OF ANTIBODIES AND VACCINES TO PROTECT.

1. In all people with antibodies to the AIDS virus, some virus persists in brain and other cells from which it cannot be removed. In contrast to most virus infections, antibodies to a lentivirus do not provide protective immunity; they fail to neutralize or eliminate it. Although many people infected with the AIDS virus look and feel well for several years, destruction of the cells of the brain and immune systems is progressing slowly.

2. The outlook for a successful vaccine is bleak. None is available for lentivirus diseases of animals. Search for a vaccine against infectious anemia of horses for eight years, and against maedi-visna in sheep for forty years has proved futile. Indeed when antibodies to a lentivirus are produced artificially by vaccination, animals die after subsequent infection more rapidly than those which are not. In spite of many successful vaccines, it should be realized that for the majority of viral and bacterial diseases, vaccines do not work.

D. BLEAK OUTLOOK FOR A CURE.

1. No simple, effective, curative drug, like penicillin will be available for AIDS in the foreseeable future, because once a person is infected, the viral genetic code is permanently inserted into the human genetic code of cells in the brain and other tissues. Any drug which blocks replication of the virus will have to be taken for life. All drugs used so

far are highly toxic and expensive. If a cheap, apparently effective drug becomes available it will take several decades to be certain that it is both safe and effective. Nevertheless, many companies will announce "promising new drugs and a "breakthrough" in the treatment for AIDS for simple commercial motives.

2. The handling of recent AZT clinical trials by the U.S. Government was particularly important. The U.S. Public Health Service insisted the trials cease long before any long term benefit of the drug had been shown, and before the manufacturing company suggested it, thereby misleading the public into believing a "cure" for AIDS was already in the pipeline. Such disinformation weakens the political will to implement tough control measures required to halt the spread of the virus.

E. TRANSMISSION OF AIDS—SEXUAL INTERCOURSE.

1. Scientists and doctors have repeatedly stated as fact that the AIDS virus is fundamentally transmitted during sexual intercourse, but is, unfortunately, sometimes transmitted in blood. This is highly misleading, though published laboratory and epidemiological evidence, and editorials in scientific and medical journals, have been heavily slanted to support this "fact."

2. In reality, AIDS is characteristically a blood transmitted infection, which is only transmitted with difficulty during sexual intercourse compared with the genuine sexually transmitted diseases, gonorrhea and trichomonosias. All the exceptional epidiomological evidence is consistent with this view.

3. Obviously AIDS is transmittable during sexual inter-

course, but so is influenza, glandular fever and scabies. Sexual intercourse is only one of many ways by which the virus can be transmitted, and is by no means the most efficient.

4. The illusion that AIDS is essentially a sexually transmitted disease arose from the first observations that AIDS appeared to affect only sodomites with numerous partners. However, sodomy is not sexual intercourse in the biological sense of the word. As we are dealing with a very important biological event, the transmission of a lethal parasite from one human host to another, it is essential that scientists use words describing the transmission with the utmost precision.

5. In biological terms sexual intercourse means the union of male and female which may result in reproduction of the species. In mammals, this invariably requires contact between male and female genitals. Consequently sexual intercourse between two men in the biological sense is impossible.

6. Scientists who state, or simply imply sodomy is sexual intercourse without some qualification are being imprecise and misleading, whether intentionally or not.

7. Homosexual men engaged in homosexual activities frequently insert their fingers, fist, penis or tongue into the lower intestinal tract of their partners. These maneuvers transmit any virus which persists in the blood for months or years with devastating efficiency, even though no virus is present in either semen or saliva. This has been shown very clearly with hepatitis B virus which, in prosperous communities, infects the majority of homosexual men within three years of becoming sexually active; whereas hepatitis B infec-

tion remains rare among heterosexual men and women, even though they frequently change partners.

F. DISINFORMATION FROM SCIENTISTS.

1. The AIDS virus persists in an infectious state (i.e. cell-free virus) in blood and semen levels up to 25,000 virions per milliliter, according to the only published paper giving this critically important information. Cell-free virions were detected easily in saliva over two years ago, but quantitative studies have still not been published.*

2. No infectious virion has been detected in semen, according to the only two detailed studies published on the subject, which between them included a grand total of three men examined. In ten percent of fifty infected men, according to another report sent to me personally but which gave few details, cell-associated virus has been detected in a few white blood cells in semen, but never in spermatozoa.

3. Virions have been detected in the vaginal secretions in only trivial quantities—about one millilitre—indicating that their infectivity is minimal.

4. The scale of deception and misinformation perpetrated by virologists, clinicians, editors of scientific and medical journals about the infectivity of genital secretions, compared with that of blood, serum and saliva, has been astonishing. In the presence of a new, lethal virus spreading amongst people for which no vaccine or cure is in sight, every sane person would assume that scientists have

* Why not? How much longer will the World Health Organization and the U.S. medical fraternity insist that kissing, where saliva is exchanged, cannot be a means of AIDS transmission? How many innocent people must be sacrificed before our medical institutions are forced to tell the truth?

been working flat out to verify precisely how it is transmitted.

5. On the contrary, having assumed for a variety of motives that AIDS is a sexually transmitted disease like syphilis or gonorrhea, a negligible research effort has gone into the critical matter of transmission. A few preliminary papers were published and their findings have been frequently quoted as showing the opposite of what is actually showed. When this is pointed out in letters to the editors of major medical and scientific journals, publication has been refused. No attempt has been made to check, double-check, and recheck findings in other laboratories, and in other countries, to rectify published errors.

6. As far as it goes, the tiny research effort into infectivity of bodily fluids indicates that saliva is far more infectious than genital secretions, but that blood and serum is vastly more infectious than either. Consequently the idea that condoms can have any significant effect on the spread of AIDS in a nation is utterly preposterous.

7. Governments all over the world are spending millions of pounds advising their citizens to prevent AIDS by using condoms on the basis of manifestly fraudulent misrepresentation of scientific evidence presented by scientists themselves.*

8. The AIDS virus is unusually stable outside the human body. It retains almost all of its infectivity after seven days in water at room temperature and sometimes after being kept dry for a week. A virus with this degree of stability,

* This strong statement by a world-renowned AIDS specialist shows all too well one of the biggest—and deadliest—lies told by government and the medical profession to the American people about the use of condoms being safely preventive measure against AIDS.

which persists in the blood and is shed in saliva, cannot possibly fail to be transmitted in many ways apart from sexual intercourse.

G. VARIABLE EFFICIENCY IN MEANS OF TRANSMISSION.

1. A virus which persists in moderate quantities in the blood for years and is shed through saliva will be transmitted with far greater ease by some means than by others.

2. Injection of the virus through the skin in hypodermic needles is the most certain way of transmission. This happens when blood-contaminated hypodermics are reused without sterilization, as is common among drug addicts in the West and in health care facilities in less prosperous countries. It also occurs when virus-contaminated blood transfusions and clotting factors are administered.

3. Male homosexual contact of the finger, penis or tongue with the rectal wall of another male transmits the virus very easily. Seventy percent of the male homosexual population of San Francisco became infected within six years of the arrival of the virus in the city, and nearly thirty percent of London homosexuals are already infected. The percentages are rising remoreselessly in large cities throughout the Western world, unaffected by the highly acclaimed "safe sex" propaganda.

4. Well over fifty percent of newborn babies of infected mothers are infected.

5. Moderately efficient means of transmission include mouth-to-mouth and genital contact before and during normal sexual intercourse, oral salivary contact between

small children, needle stick injuries to nursing staff, and chance contact of sores or abrasions with blood, serum and saliva or sputum.*

6. Inefficient means of transmission include social kissing, inhalation of respiratory aerosols caused by coughing or sneezing and blood-sucking insects.†

7. Transmission by inhalation is only inefficient because of the relatively small number of virions shed in saliva and bronchial secretions. However, if an AIDS virion is inhaled into the lung, it is engulfed by an amoeba-like macrophage on the lining of the alvoli (air sacs). It has been shown repeatedly in the laboratory that the AIDS virus readily infects people by this route.

8. Understandably, and wisely, the Department of Health and Social Services has officially advised all British dental surgeons to always wear masks to avoid AIDS virus infection when using high speed drills. These drills make aerosols of saliva, similar to those produced by sneezing.

9. Chronic lymphoid intestinal pneumonia is a well-recognized variety of pneumonia caused directly by infection of the lungs with the AIDS virus. It is similar to the pneumonia of maedi-visna in sheep and is particularly common in children with AIDS. When associated with pulmonary

* At the time Dr. Seale made this report, the civilian medical community was not yet knowledgeable about the role of Denditric cells and Langerhan cells in AIDS transmission. That was still secret information inside the Chemical and Bacteriological warfare labs. Had Dr. Seale known then what we know now, he would have presumably included close skin contact, even with no sores or abrasions present.

† Since Dr. Seale wrote this report, it has been firmly established that surgeon's operating tools, such as high-speed drills, can and do throw out a fine aerosol spray of blood.

tuberculosis, a very common complication of AIDS, it is inevitable that coughing will produce some aerosols containing tubercule bacilli and the AIDS virus. After a fluid in the aerosols evaporates, the minute dry flakes containing tubercule and AIDS virus float around in the air indefinitely and remain infectious for days.

10. The normal route of transmission of the maedi-visna lentivirus between adult sheep is by respiratory aerosols when they are crowded closely together in winter shelters. Maedi-visna is not a sexually transmitted disease of sheep.

11. The efficiency of transmission of AIDS virus by biting insects will depend upon the quantity of virions in the blood of the bitten person, the anatomical structure of the biting parts of the insects, their feeding habits and other factors.

The AIDS virus has been shown to remain highly infectious in the stomach of a bed-bug for at least two hours. It has been shown that it can infect the cells of insects, including mosquitoes and cockroaches both in laboratory cell cultures and in live insects. Replication of the virus in the insect has not been demonstrated.

H. SATURATION OF THE BRITISH POPULATION WITH THE VIRUS.

1. There is a key to estimating how long it will take for the people of Great Britain to be saturated with AIDS virus, if its spread is allowed to continue unchecked as at present. This is the application of probability theory to the known facts about the virus, its pathogenesis, the frequency of "contact" and the efficiency with which different "contacts" transmit the virus.

2. The basic facts are that the entire population is susceptible to infection, and once people are infected, they remain potentially infectious to others for life.

3. As the number of people infected rises, the probability of transmission during any contact between people also rises.

4. Initially the virus was introduced into Britain from the United States by homosexual men who soon infected others by having frequent, efficient "contacts"—sodomy with strangers. As the number of infected homosexuals rises, the probability of infection being transmitted through one "contact" rises at first exponentially, but then a slower doubling rate saturation point with the homosexual population is approached.

5. As numbers of infected homosexuals and addicts increase, efficient "contacts" rarely performed—such as receiving a blood transfusion, or clotting factor or having a baby—infect more and more people.

6. Once a critical mass of people has been created by the highly efficient "contacts," then "contacts" which are only moderately efficient, but occur frequently—such as normal sexual intercourse or small children playing together—will spread the virus in ever-widening circles throughout the population.

7. Finally, highly inefficient "contacts" which occur very frequently, such as coughing in public and being bitten by insects will infect many people as millions of infected persons interact with the non-infected, and saturation of the entire British population becomes unstoppable.

I. GROUPS MISINFORMING THE PUBLIC AND THEIR MOTIVES.

A. Homosexual men.

1. Homosexual men have been the most determined and effective in distorting the truth about AIDS.

2. They have been so effective because there is a scattering of homosexuals amongst all the key professional groups involved, scientists, doctors, medical editors, journalists, lawyers, politicians and priests.

3. The initial impact of AIDS on homosexuals in the West inevitably resulted in an unusually high proportion of them becoming involved in the disease since it first surfaced. Many of the men who are particularly knowledgeable about and dedicated to AIDS research, treatment, legislation, publication and education are homosexuals.

4. Most in the professions are only identifiable as homosexuals to other men with similar tastes—a few have "come out" and even the wives of those who are married are usually unaware of their habits. Hence they automatically form a type of secret society without even trying, with wide ramifications across professional, institutional and national boundaries.

5. Homosexual men have been vectors of the virus throughout the Western world and if it had not been for their activities, very few people in prosperous countries would now be infected. Their oft-repeated statement that they are the major victims of the virus is true, but it is also true that they have spread the virus to each other by their practices and thence onward to the rest of the population.

6. Many do not want to face reality because of guilt, most do not wish to change their ways and a few seeing death and

destruction facing themselves and their friends are dedicated to destroying the rest of society with them.

7. All wish to deny the reality that restricting the freedom of homosexuals to infect each other and other people is essential if our society is not to be destroyed by the virus.

B. Scientists.

1. Every biological scientist who has dispassionately studied the virus and the epidemic knows that the origins of the virus could lie in the development of modern biology, just as the origins of the nuclear bomb with modern physics.

2. Most biological scientists have not yet come to terms with the terrible truth and have developed various neurotic reactions to cope with it.

3. Many have developed a selective denial of reality and genuinely cannot see what is happening. Most who see it keep quiet, but increasing numbers are talking privately, though they still lack the moral courage to speak out in public. They still hope it is a nightmare which will vanish with tomorrow's dawn.

4. Some who know perfectly well what is happening are deliberately fudging scientific data to keep the heat off them and fellow scientists of their molecular biological "club."*

C. Editors of Scientific and Medical Journals.

1. Medical and scientific editors have misled their professional colleagues about the nature and severity of the AIDS epidemic for five years. By selective acceptances or rejection

---

* What Dr. Seale is telling us here, very gingerly, is that the truth about the genesis of AIDS is well known to scientists and virologists, but fear has sealed their lips. They are convinced that the AIDS virus was artificially created—and they understand the reason why: population control.

of original papers and letters, and by selecting authors to write "safe" editorials and review articles, they have perpetuated dangerous misconceptions.

2. As the harsh reality of what is happening becomes even more obvious, editors have adopted a range of neurotic reactions similar to those of the scientists.*

D. Doctors.

1. Most doctors are incapable of conceiving the scale of the problem, as only three hundred people have died from AIDS in Britain the last five years, but 20,000 have died of cancer of the lung. How can AIDS be that important?

2. An epidemic slow virus disease is new to medical science and its significance largely incomprehensible to doctors, because it is outside of both their practical experience and theoretical training.

3. Epidemics were supposed to have been abolished along with old fever hospitals and TB sanatoria twenty-five years ago. It is difficult to change cherished beliefs. It is assumed that scientists will soon have a vaccine and the AIDS epidemic will disappear like bad flu epidemics.

4. Doctors who have treated many patients with AIDS are profoundly shocked at their own and modern medicine's inability to restore the health of so many young patients. Although death be delayed, remissions are temporary. Deterioration is so protracted, often lasting years, that many AIDS patients kill themselves as a means of escape.

---

* Under this heading is the classic example, an article in the American Medical News: "AIDISM, a New Form of Discrimination." Its thrust was that those infected with AIDS have a greater right than those who are not infected and who wish to remain AIDS-free.

5. Many young doctors working only on AIDS patients soon become depressed themselves. The term "AIDS burn-out" is now widely used in America; it has similarities with wartime battle exhaustion.

6. Many senior doctors in charge of numerous AIDS patients develop profoundly neurotic attitudes which enable them to cope with their job by selective denial of reality. In support of their patients for whom they can do so little medically, they fiercely defend their right of confidentiality and freedom of association, totally ignoring public health responsibility to ensure that others are not infected. They are regularly consulted by Government and the Media and other doctors on how to control the epidemic.

E. Journalists.

1. In the face of a lethal disease, journalists and the media editors have been frightened to contradict the conventional wisdom being put across by the scientists. There have been no serious attempts at investigative journalism into the wealth of scientific scandals surrounding AIDS.

2. They have often given way to tremendous pressure put upon them by scientists and homosexuals to understate the seriousness of the epidemic and, in the last two years, have capitulated to demands that AIDS be portrayed as an 'ordinary' venereal disease.

3. Understandably, as in war that is going badly, all news of breakthroughs with cures and vaccines is given lavish cover. These lull politicians and public into fatal inaction.

F. Politicians.

1. Leading politicians from all parties in all nations have, until recently, hardly mentioned AIDS in public. Accepting the earlier views of scientists that it is just a homosexual

disease, and the revised view that it is only a venereal disease, they know that taking AIDS seriously would have gained them few votes.

2. No prominent politician has thought there was reason to doubt the much publicized opinions of scientists and public health doctors concerning the facts about AIDS.

J. VARIETIES OF MISINFORMATION.

1. People with AIDS are categorized as belonging to a small number of "risk groups," giving the false impression that the vast majority of people cannot get AIDS.

2. AIDS is portrayed as only a behavioral disease caused by sexual and narcotic misdemeanors. This implies that if anybody gets AIDS, it is their own fault.

3. Emphasis on transmission of the virus during sexual intercourse and education as a solution to the epidemic implies that the disease will disappear with modified behavior. This misses the point that as the epidemic explodes, infection by chance, non-sexual, contact becomes even more common.

4. By equating sodomy with sexual intercourse, the impression is given that homosexuals have been just unlucky to get infected before heterosexuals. In reality homosexual activity has spread the virus throughout the population at a vastly greater speed than normal sexual intercourse could achieve.

5. The value of blood tests for diagnoses of AIDS virus infection is repeatedly denigrated by those who do not want them introduced compulsorily. In fact the blood test is an unusually reliable diagnostic tool.

6. The suffering of those with AIDS is highlighted while ignoring the sufferings of those who will get AIDS in

the future if appropriate steps are not taken to stop its spread.

7. The rights of those infected with the virus are stressed while the rights of the uninfected to be protected from infection with a lethal virus are ignored and glossed over. Protection of the life of its citizens is the major obligation of the State.

8. Misinformation is perpetuated by homosexuals actively obstructing the publication, in the scientific, or general press of facts and conclusions which they want suppressed.

K. METHOD OF CONTROL.

1. The most urgent step to be taken is to break the pervasive grip by homosexuals on the information and disinformation which has emanated for so long from journals of science and medicine. Once this has been done, other scientists, doctors, politicians can stress accurately the reality of the situation.

2. Once the truth is known and published, the steps to be taken to halt the epidemic become more obvious and less controversial.

3. Speed is the essence because every day that is lost will increase the human misery which in any event will be vast.

4. We are facing a national catastrophe equal to any in the history of our nation. The life of every citizen is at stake. Death from AIDS is a protracted horror unequaled by other diseases.

5. The only way to halt the spread of the virus is to identify all those who are infected by compulsory testing. Government must then take whatever steps are required to ensure that those infected do not pass the virus to anyone else.

6. The longer this action is delayed the greater will be the task when it is finally undertaken and the greater the danger that the spread of the virus will then be unstoppable.

7. The actions required of Government are comparable to those taken in waging a war of survival.

8. The war against AIDS is a war of survival. If we lose, Britain and all her people perish.

That's the end of Dr. Seale's memorandum. Everything he said applies with equal force to America.

APPENDIX B

In September of 1983, one hundred and fifteen virologists from around the world met in secret sessions at Cold Spring Harbor. Not one single word from that conference has ever been published, but according according to intelligence sources, the role of viruses was fully discussed in relation to biological warfare against the civilian population. It was stressed that an organism as simple as a virus could threaten the very existence of all human life on earth.

Here is the first sketchy outline of what those virologists secretly shared with each other at Cold Spring Harbor in 1983:

HIV genetic information is filed in the form of ribonucleic acid (RNA), the opposite of most other organisms which have genetic material comprising deoxyribonucleic acid (DNA.) DNA carries the information, strung together like molecular beads, that is critical to the organism. Scientists were now finding out that molecules are made of matter, whose origin the proponents of the "big-bang" theory cannot explain; these molecules being the building blocks of the universe.

The sequence of molecular "beads" are then mirrored in plants and animals. The "mirrored" image is in fact RNA, and in it are the information codes needed to make proteins—the life-giving component of living organisms. The strings are then "beaded" with smaller molecules called amino acids. In this manner most organisms produce their own proteins, but this does not happen in the case of viruses, which are parasites and must have a host to live off.

At the Cold Spring Harbor conference, it was stated that viruses do not have a life-like bacteria; a virus is an incomplete cell, because its genetic material is incomplete and is covered by a hard shell of protein. Before a virus can "live," it has to latch onto and invade living cells. When it penetrates the host cell, it then comes alive and begins to replicate. In the case of the HIV virus, the replication process is extremely rapid.

AIDS-HIV viruses have RNA as their genetic material. By inserting its RNA into the host cell, the cell is deceived into stepping up its manufacture of viral proteins. Part of these proteins are the enzymes needed to synthethize more viral DNA. It is from this process that the term "Retro" (backward) was coined because the host cell is deceived, like the mother bird who feeds the baby cuckoo in her nest. The host cell is blinded into believing it must convert viral RNA from the invader virus back to DNA. Ordinarily the cell would make RNA from DNA, but here the process is reversed. This goes on until the cell "blooms" or "flowers" with its packed HIV parasites, and the component parts burst out into the bloodstream, infecting it with millions more HIV viruses.

When the HIV virus and the healthy cell come together, the HIV receptor fuses with the membranes of the cell it is taking over. The enzyme released is known as a reverse transcriptase. This is unique to retroviruses and is totally absent in human cells. The viral RNA then enters and integrates itself in the DNA of the cell it has taken over. Once inside, the viral DNA becomes dormant, which is the period we know as the latency period. This latency period in AIDS is known to last up to ten years, but in the case of blacks and Hispanics, the HIV virus seems to have a far shorter latency period and acts in a more virulent manner toward the host cell.*

At some time during the latency period, the virus will be triggered. Russian scientists had apparently perfected a technique using electromagnetic signals on the same wavelength as the virus, which, when "radiated" by the signals, would spring to life. A viral "Manchurian Candidate," so to speak. More common causes are believed to be repeated occurrences of infections, such as of Hepatitus B or herpes, for example.

The manufacture of viral proteins and viral DNA—the two main components of HIV—is stimulated. Next comes the "flowering" or "budding." At this point, the victim will be at great risk and a danger to all who come into contact with him or her. With "budding," the HIV virus takes part of the outer fatty cell membrane and its glycoprotein (molecules of sugar) and swallows them up.

What's most diabolical about HIV is that it prefers to attack cells in human bodies assigned the task of protecting the body from any and all foreign invaders, the so-called T-4 cells.

* Notice that they were discussing more than a decade ago that the HIV virus attacked blacks and Hispanics with greater frequency and more virulence than it attacked whites. Have you ever seen that information in the media?

APPENDIX C

What follows here are lengthy quotes from an internal Cold Springs Harbor document and a government intelligence report. The first reads as though it is written by a knowledgeable researcher "briefing" a recent arrival—perhaps his new boss—and bringing him up to speed on some of the lab's work. Presumably one scientist to another. Certainly a writer and an audience who were intimately familiar with complex, scientific language.

If you're not a virologist or a microbiologist, this is extremely difficult reading. But it is worth the effort. If you will read it carefully and absorb it, and then read it again and absorb it again, the picture will gradually come into focus. Rather like watching an old Polaroid snapshot developing itself. At first it's a blank. Then there are dim outlines. And then the picture emerges. You can see exactly what you were meant (or, in this case, not meant) to see.

The second document, the intelligence report—part of which I quoted in Chapter Thirteen—speaks for itself. Read it and weep.

* * *

This is what they were writing to each other years ago at Cold Spring Harbor:

"The work done by Bang and Koprowski on mouse macrophages show the factors affecting the capacity to support replication of hepatitis viruses of an appropriate strain that killed adult mice. Peritoneal macrophages from mice able to support multiplication of the virus was noticed in some, whereas macrophages from resistant mice did not, and it follows that the resistance genes are followed through F2 and later generations, the susceptibility to support virus replication is paralleled by the macrophage susceptibility to support virus replication. Anthropod-borne viruses, West Nile and Yellow Fever (B group) show the same thing.

"For this purpose we are especially interested in genetic factors which are manifested in immunocompetent cells, namely the capacity of immunocompetent cells to react against infections and prevent their spread or to prevent development of tumors.

"The work done by the other groups is reflected in 'The Distribution of Human Blood and Other Polymorphisms' by A. F. Mourat. Here we find that there is a correlation between the geographically determined distribution characteristics of immunological importance and susceptibility to resist particular diseases. The Fy allele of the Duffy blood group is common among Negroes, while it very rarely, if ever, occurs in whites.

"Our military-related research establishments monitor microbial environment in every area of the world. Their archives store viruses and bacteria from all areas and all countries, even as we do. Like us, they are constantly adding new varieties and strains with the purpose of studying both incidence and methods of transmission. Naturally, this has to be done without attracting attention. We now know that the sudden onset of an influenza strain in 1977 that had not existed anywhere since 1951, was the cause of the 1977 epidemic. This could, and most probably did, result from experimental work carried out by such military-related research establishments.*

"The Histocompatability Group under the World Health Organization and the International Union of Immunological Societies has made a large number of studies which cover the tremendous genetic variability in the detailed structure of major histocompatibility complex (MHC) gives rise to the belief that there are viruses that preferentially affect humans with specific MHC types.†

"What we have done at Cold Spring Harbor is to examine these glycoprotein molecules to ascertain why they play a decisive part in immune system-recognition and reaction to foreign material entering the body. The unique cooperation and collaboration internationally between an as-yet limited number of microbiologists and researchers has brought forth much information concerning race and geographical location and their lymphocyte reaction with standard HL-A sera in patterns strikingly different from the cells of Caucasians studied thus far, as we found in our New Guinea studies.

* Remember the 1977 flu epidemic? It was serious enough to be treated as an ongoing story in the national news media. Is it too fantastic to suggest that the epidemic might have been created in our own Chemical and Bacteriological Warfare labs? Not if you worked at Cold Spring Harbor. They figured that's what happened.

† MHC is a genetically coded set of glycoprotein molecules located on the surface of immune system cells—the T-cells.

"There are now plans to expand this work on a much larger scale, and we shall probably see this within the next 10-12 years as part of a global orientation. Work is being carried out by such pioneers in HLA as J. Dausset of the University of Paris. As we know from the conference which took place at Evian, France in 1972, there exists a vast difference in frequencies and definitions of the HLA antigens in various racial groups."*

Here is what our intelligence agencies were reporting almost a decade ago:

"A vast international MHC-type research effort is now in motion all over the world, in particular work has been concentrated on role of macrophages as a barrier to the spread of infection and especially to find out why certain viruses are quickly taken up by machrophages. At Cold Spring Harbor the thrust of such research is to discover how macrophages may be used by the AIDS virus to spread to the rest of the body and disseminate infection.

"Funding for this rather large increase in the number of research facilities engaged in MHC-HLS studies is done by the descendants of those who were responsible for funding the Eugenics Records Office, which experiments began as far back as 1904. Molecular biology is considered by these funding

---

* This information alone would seem to confirm Samuel Evans' charges to Congress that there is a strain of AIDS virus designed to attack blacks and other "colored" races.

This author's belief that "within the next 10-12 years," histocompatibility (HLA) would expand globally has proven accurate. There have been several detailed studies of racial and geographical distributions of susceptibility to viruses.

groups as an extension of racial eugenics begun in 1904, and the work at Cold Spring Harbor reflects the continuity of detailed and sophisticated laboratory research by microbiologists to shed light on the differences in racial capabilities to resist or to succumb to virally-induced diseases.

"In 1986 there was a further gathering of the initiated at Cold Spring Harbor to hear Professor W. Bodmer of the Imperial Cancer Research Institute, a world-renowned Oxford geneticist, speak on 'The Molecular Biology of Homo Sapiens.' Behind closed doors several delegates expressed the view that population explosion was the greatest threat to the stability of the world, echoing the words of Sir Julian Huxley at the 1982 Cold Spring Harbor Conference-'world population growth is the most alarming problem and loss of genetic quality must be reversed.'

"Professor Bodmer began his address by saying: "Analyses of normal human variability in facial features, character and mental abilities is surely one of the real challenges of human genetics. Now, with the availability of polymorphic DNA markers, there is a well-defined approach. The DNA technology that is now available should in due course be able to answer the question as to whether indeed the genes that control facial features and certain aspects of behavior are closely linked . . . Knowledge of the total human genome sequence has profound implications, not only for the analysis, prevention, and treatment of disease, but also for the better understanding of normal variations, and through that, hopefully, making a contribution to solving broader problems of society.

"Behind closed doors, Bodmer left his listeners in no doubt that one of the greatest 'broader problems of society' was overpopulation of the world by 'undesirables,' and population explosions among black nations urgently needed to be arrested and stopped altogether, and their populations drastically reduced. The sum and substance of Bodmer's remarks left his audience in no doubt that genetically-engineered retroviruses were the only hope of achieving the desired goal."